SEVEN PLANES OF
EXISTENCE

SEVEN PLANES OF EXISTENCE
The Philosophy of the ThetaHealing® Technique

VIANNA STIBAL
Creator of the ThetaHealing® Technique

HAY HOUSE

Carlsbad, California • New York City
London • Sydney • New Delhi

Published in the United States by: Hay House LLC: www.hayhouse.com®
Published in Australia by: Hay House Australia Publishing Pty Ltd: www.hayhouse.com.au
Published in the United Kingdom by: Hay House UK Ltd: www.hayhouse.co.uk
Published in India by: Hay House Publishers (India) Pvt Ltd: www.hayhouse.co.in

Cover and interior design: Leanne Siu Anastasi
Interior images: Shutterstock/Thinkstock

Originally published by Hay House UK, 978-1-78180-545-9

Library of Congress Control Number: 2015935172

Tradepaper ISBN: 978-1-4019-4855-9

18 17 16 15 14 13 12 11 10 9
1st edition, January 2016

Printed in the United States of America

This product uses responsibly sourced papers and/or recycled materials.
For more information, see www.hayhouse.com.

Storm the Gates of Heaven!

As the maelstrom of life besets me,
I kneel, my head bent.
From every direction,
From within, from without,
I am besieged by darkness.
Flooded with dark emotions,
I feel the suffering of fear, doubt and despair.
I feel the frustration of limitations.
I feel desire and love, melancholy and elation.
I feel fleeting joy and it is gone.

The realization awakens,
Of the intense anguish of mortality,
Of the light that I am, so brief and fleeting,
And of all that would extinguish my soul.

From inside comes the thunder of defiance.
Reverberating through my soul, the power builds,
And I become self-aware.

Resolute against all the forces that would assail me,
Against all the vicissitudes of the evil within and outside me,
In the heart of desolation,
Within the blackness that would consume me,
I awaken and kindle the light within.

For the first time, I can see what holds me.
My body is anchored to this Earth,
I am chained as Prometheus,
Held with invisible fetters,
Shaped by children of a lesser God.
I begin my struggle to be free,
Gnashing at my shackles,
As Fenrir the wolf.

I find the acceptance of the bitter and sweet.
From every pore of my being,
I begin to bleed,
To cry a river against the bitterness of despair,
Shedding tears of liquid resolve that wash me clean.
I search for the center, and find the equilibrium.

In the agony of life, I learn acceptance.
I surrender completely, and look up.
From my knees, I rise to my feet,
Breaking the chains of fear
With the pure energy of thought.
An explosion of blue light
Dissolves the invisible fetters,
For I fear death no more,
And beginning from within,
I become the microcosm.

All becomes clear, and I see that I stand,
Within the Vortex of life,
The Vortex that binds me and holds me to this life.
It swirls about me and above me,
A mighty pillar that leads to the sky,
And beyond, into infinity.

Gathering the power about me,
From the magic that is pure,
I roar as the power builds,
Against time, against death, against fear and despair,
Making them an illusion.
I will escape.
I will be free.
I will *become*
A being of the combined elements,
I will *become*

The Philosopher's Stone, the macrocosm,
I will *become*
The phoenix from the ashes,
Ascending from this corporal prison,
Screaming the name of the Creator,
Coursing with the power of divinity,
Suffused with illumination,
Rising as a storm toward the cosmos,
To assail the Gates of Heaven!

I will storm the Gates of Heaven.
Without hope, I will charge the Gates,
To break myself upon them,
To spend the essence of my soul,
To witness them fall before me,
Or let every atom of my being explode in the endeavor,
To break free from karma,
Or cease to exist, and be no more.

Armed with the Spear of my Belief,
I ascend beyond the universe,
Through radiances immeasurable,
To reach a barrier of color and vibration
That seeks to bar my way.
But I will not be denied!
I will become the Planes of Existence!

Each plane becomes integrated within me,
And with the power of thought,
I will speak the *Word* to the universe,
The *Word* that becomes an intonation,
The intonation, a pulsation of sound,
A frequency so powerful it *cannot be denied*,
The force expanding as it assails the Gates,
With the power of a thousand exploding stars.

The timeless Gates begin to vibrate and shriek,
And explode in a burst of golden light.

Then comes the vibration,
The intonation of divine sound,
Coming from the heart of heaven,
The voice of a multitude of angels,
Becoming the very voice of God,
Rushing toward me and I toward it,
Speaking with one voice, one query.
In tears of joy,
In exultation,
I open to the question:

'Child of man,
Is there resolve within you,
To go beyond the Gates of Heaven,
To touch the face of God,
And step beyond, to be as one,
With the Creator of All That Is?
Here, then, is what you seek!
Hearken, and greet the All That Is!
Open yourself, little spark of God,
And know divinity!
Welcome to the Creator of All That Is.'

I rise into a brilliant pearlescent pillar of light,
That encompasses me,
That makes me complete, whole.
I become light,
No longer separate from Creation,
But becoming Creation itself.

GUY STIBAL, DECEMBER 2006

We are all looking for the Gates to Heaven. Whether we are rich or poor, agnostic or religious, deep in our heart we all hope they exist – a portal to a life beyond this one, to a higher consciousness ... and, for those who believe, to God.

The Gates to Heaven are the barriers made of our beliefs that separate us from a loving God.

Perhaps if the Gates of our beliefs burst asunder, we will know God in this mortal body. Perhaps it is as Meister Eckhart says, that God does not exist without us, nor us without God.

This is how I perceive Vianna. She and others like her are here to open the Gates of Heaven and keep them open, so that there is no separation between a loving God and us.

The planes of existence give all of us the road map to storm the Gates of Heaven.

CONTENTS

INTRODUCTION

In this book, information will be revealed from one of the most powerful energy-healing techniques, ThetaHealing®. ThetaHealing is a process of meditation that we believe creates physical, psychological, and spiritual healing using the Theta brainwave. While in a pure Theta state of mind, we are able to connect to the Creator of All That Is through focused prayer.

It is through the Creator of All That Is that I learned how to create physical healing, progress spiritually, and find a path to enlightenment. ThetaHealing was born and proved its validation to me through what I believe to be the spontaneous healing of my leg. I am still coming to an understanding of how important this first healing and learning experience was to me and how it will continue to be important to people interested in this work long after I have left this life and moved to a higher place. That spontaneous healing was the tiny seed that grew into the sacred tree of ThetaHealing.

This is a companion to my first two books, *ThetaHealing* and *Advanced ThetaHealing*. In *ThetaHealing*, I explain the step-by-step processes of the ThetaHealing reading, healing, belief work, feeling work, digging work, and gene work, and give an introduction to the planes of existence and additional knowledge for the beginner. In *Advanced ThetaHealing*, I give a short description of my experiences with each plane of existence and how to use them in healing with the mind. These two books give the reader an in-depth guide to belief, feeling, digging, and gene work, insights into the planes of existence, and the beliefs that I believe are essential for spiritual evolution. The focus of these books is teaching how to access healing abilities from the Seventh Plane of Existence by using the unconditional love of the Creator of All That Is.

This book does not include many of the specific step-by-step processes that proliferate in my first two books, but it is necessary to reach an understanding of these processes in order to utilize this book fully.

In this book, I will take you to dimensions that I believe to be the beginnings of life itself, on a journey that leads outward past the universe and offers the concept that in a Theta state of mind it is possible to connect to divine energy *before* it becomes anything in this universe. I will explain the planes of existence, which provide us with a conceptual framework for understanding how and why creation works on the physical and spiritual levels, and how this relates to us on all levels of our being: mentally, spiritually, psychically, physically, and emotionally.

It is important that the concept of the planes of existence is understood, because it is the definitive philosophical guide to the art of ThetaHealing.

It is interesting to note that it took many years to compile the information about ThetaHealing into the books that people enjoy today. Inspiration for such a thing is dependent upon many factors, but mainly these books have come from years of meditation, prayer, faith, and divine guidance. This book alone took several years of considered channeling that began in a blinding flash of light when I was in Croatia, driving toward the birthplace of Nikola Tesla. This flash of light was the spark of inspiration that opened my senses and it continued coming to me in my cabin high in the mountains of Idaho. The rest of the inspiration came from you, dear reader, for without your vibration of love, this philosophy would not have come in.

We all have different motivation for learning something like ThetaHealing. Some people are searching for knowledge, some are merely curious, and others have less than altruistic motives. But the majority of people who learn it are pure of heart and seeking to expand abilities that are lying dormant in their mind. This is what ThetaHealing is designed to do: teach people how to harness their psychic abilities through spiritual awareness. I began in much the same way and I guess you could say that ThetaHealing started because I needed to control my own psychic abilities.

What first motivated me to do this was watching the struggles that my mother went through. I perceive my mother as a great psychic soul essence poured into a fanatically religious woman who can't keep it contained. Her religious beliefs are at odds with her inner essence and for many years she fought her intuition because she considered it to be wrong, immoral, or even evil, because of bigotry and superstition. Now she does use it from time to time, but because of what she's been taught, she always questions it, wondering if this beautiful essence is coming from a dark place. Had she been able to accept it as a gift from God, however, she would have been able to let it fly free, unfettered as a soaring falcon that views creation from the clouds.

When I was 15 years old, I became aware of the same psychic essence inside myself. Between the ages of 17 and 27, I couldn't control it at all. It was only when I was 31 that I began to control it instead of it controlling me. This meant that instead of receiving spurts of psychic information or being haunted by spirits and other energies, I learned how to focus and deal with what was happening. If the spirits were negative, I told them to go away. Sometimes they would and other times they'd come back. But then I learned to send them to God's light, and they stayed there.

I learned how to do this through guidance from my 'heavenly father.' One of the most important things that I learned from the religious side of mother was that there was a heavenly father who loved me and whom I could talk to whenever I wanted. From three years old, I began to have conversations with him. The answers to my questions weren't always what I wanted, but I always got an answer.

Some years later it was through this relationship with my heavenly father that I was introduced to the Laws of the universe. This began with a visionary experience when I met the Law of Truth from the Sixth Plane of Existence in my living room. This Law showed me that I was creating difficult situations in my life due to my belief systems *and that I could manifest changes through a connection to the divine.*

This was a profound experience, but the reason I had it was because I'd asked for it and on some level I'd believed it was possible. The reason I'd believed this was because when I was a small child my mother used to read to me from the Bible about a man named Solomon. Solomon asked

God for one thing, and that one thing was wisdom. This story stuck in my mind even as an adult. I believed I could ask God for one thing, and I spent hours thinking about what that one thing should be.

What one thing would help me take care of my family? I had just opened a business doing psychic readings, so I asked God to show me *truth*. If I could tell people the truth in a reading, they'd come back for another reading and would tell others about me. They might not like me personally, but if I could tell them the truth then I'd be doing them a service anyway. So I asked to see truth, but I had no idea that the Law of Truth would show up in my living room!

Since that time, the Law of Truth has been the Law that I've been most affiliated with. It still comes to visit me from time to time, curious, I think, to see how I'm progressing with my life challenges.

After this experience, I was on a quest to know pure truth, to know and communicate with the highest divinity, and to know how the universe was created.

It was about this time that people first asked me to teach classes. As I started to do so, my students became my motivation to stop and think about what I was doing psychically, to understand it, and to see if others could do it as well. This was the beginning of my understanding of the seven planes of existence. I saw a need for this understanding in my students too. They needed the balance this provided.

This led me to ask the Creator to show me the constructs of the universe. However, the information didn't come to me all at once. My brain had to develop enough to be able to process it.

My students also wanted to know more about the Laws, so I said to the Creator, 'I want to write a book that will show my students how to use all the Laws of the universe. Will you explain that to me?'

The answer was something I didn't expect: 'When you're ready.'

This hurt my feelings. I asked God again, but again I was told, 'You'll be given it when you're ready.'

I asked, 'What do I need in order to be ready?'

The Creator said, 'You need to learn a few things.'

In my infinite wisdom, I said, 'I know all kinds of things.'

The Creator simply repeated, 'You need to learn a few things.'

'What things do I need to learn?'

Suddenly my life went into chaos and the work that I loved so dearly was being attacked online. I couldn't understand why this was happening to me. What did I need to learn?

I got the answer when I went to a Buddhist temple in Japan.

As I related in *On the Wings of Prayer*, after teaching a class in Tokyo in 2009 I visited a 13th-century Buddhist temple and monastery called Engaku-ji, by Kamakura city. Some of the remains of the Buddha were purported to be stored in a grotto there and I wanted to experience the energy.

When I stepped up to the grotto, I felt a sharp pain in my chest, as if an electric shock had passed through my body. Then came a strange tingling, followed by the sensation of being showered with rose petals and the essence of laughter. I asked the Creator, 'What's this?' and heard, 'This is compassion.'

I felt confused, because I thought I knew what compassion felt like.

The Creator explained: 'This is what the compassion of the Buddha feels like. Everyone who has developed the virtue of true compassion has a feeling that becomes an essence of their own, and this is the compassion of the Buddha. There are many virtues that you need to acquire.'

Later I went to see the Daibutsu Buddha of Kamakura, a huge bronze statue of the Buddha in the grounds of Kotoku-in temple. There was a little shop there with many different kinds of buddha statue for sale. I asked the Creator which I should buy to represent the virtue I needed to acquire, then picked the one I felt drawn to. I expected it to be a buddha of protection, because I was being attacked on the internet. But when I asked what kind it was, I was told it was a buddha of mercy.

This disappointed me, because it was telling me that I should have mercy toward those who were making false accusations against me and those who were taken in by them. Somehow this had to be the wrong buddha. I grabbed one from a different section, but the message on the bottom was the same: 'Mercy.' I looked at some of the other statues in that section to see if they all said the same thing, but they were all different. The message was clear: somehow I had to find a way to forgive those who were attacking me. I took the buddha home and followed the message.

Later I realized I could never have channeled the planes of existence information without developing the virtues that I was reluctant to pursue: tolerance and mercy.

Once I'd learned this important lesson, I was ready to learn more. The Creator started me on an exploration of bending the Laws of the universe. This led me to a different understanding of dimensions and how they worked.

I also wanted to find out why it was that some people could perform consistent healings and others were inconsistent in the art. We are all connected to the Creator, so why should this be?

I think I have found some of the reasons for this anomaly, because I asked the Creator the right questions. One answer I received was that the people who could do healings had different thought-patterns than other people. This changed their view of reality. They didn't accept what other people defined as reality and went their own way.

Most of us don't do this. Nor do we realize that we have latent talents that are struggling to awaken inside us. We are unbelievably powerful without knowing it. We are composed of the essence of light itself. Even though we are living in a three-dimensional world, our spiritual essence is multi-dimensional in nature. When we are in a human body we act three-dimensionally, but our soul knows that there are realms beyond the physical. These realms are the seven planes of existence. I invite you to discover them through the power of a Theta thought wave while you are still in a human body.

1

THE SEVEN PLANES OF EXISTENCE

I believe that there are seven planes of existence. They are the seen and unseen forces of the cosmos that define the different dimensions of this universe and those beyond it. They are so vast that the human mind must be in an abstract state to comprehend them. The Theta state of mind enables us to perceive these inexplicable forces in all their majesty through the Creator of All That Is.

Each of the planes has its own particular energy, which is best described as a vibration. The *frequency of vibration* is what makes the planes different from one another and the spiritual and physical inhabitants of the planes different as well. The higher the frequency of vibration, the faster the atoms move. For instance, the molecules in the solid objects of the First Plane move very slowly. The molecules in the plants of the Second Plane move more quickly, and so on throughout the planes. These vibrations are the essence of life in all its forms.

The vibrational forces of the planes have both vast and tiny proportions that, once understood, can be influenced by the power of pure thought.

The planes are divided by thin veils that take the form of beliefs that are programmed into the subconscious mind of every man, woman, and child on this planet. When we go up to the Seventh Plane of Existence, we learn how to drop these veils of belief so that we can realize we are not separate from the planes but connected to all of them.

Each plane of existence is subject to its own conditions, rules, Laws, and commitments. By their very nature, the first six planes have illusions

SEVEN PLANES OF EXISTENCE

within them, but the Seventh Plane is the essence of truth and divinity.

The planes are so vast that the human mind must be in an abstract state to comprehend them and so tiny that they cannot be measured. In order to understand them, we must be in a Theta brainwave, which creates a divine state of mind. I call this a Theta state. It enables us to be receptive to the vast internal and external landscape that composes creation. And it permits us to communicate with the Creator. The way that we are able to perceive the planes of existence in all their majesty is through the Creator of All That Is of the Seventh Plane of Existence.

The Seventh Plane of Existence

This is the plane of the Creator of All That Is, the energy that flows through all things to create life. Here we have the realization that we are part of All That Is, part of God.

On the Seventh Plane, we can utilize the energies of all the planes without being bound by any oaths and commitments to them. This is because the energy of the Seventh Plane creates the other planes. It is the energy that makes the quarks that make the protons, neutrons and electrons that in turn make up the nucleus of an atom.

The Sixth Plane of Existence

This is the plane of the Laws that create the very fabric of the universe, such as the Law of Time, the Law of Magnetism, the Law of Gravity, the Law of Light, and many more.

The Fifth Plane of Existence

This is the plane of the divine and semi-divine beings, the plane of the masters, such as Jesus Christ and the Buddha. It is divided into different levels of vibration and consciousness. The lower levels are the ultimate in dualism. Everyone on this planet is some kind of Fifth-Plane being.

The Fourth Plane of Existence

This plane is the realm of spirit – what some people would call the 'spirit world.' It is where spirits exist after death, where our ancestors are in waiting. It is the school of the Fifth-Plane beings – the spirits of this place are still learning and have not graduated to higher vibrations of reality.

The Third Plane of Existence

This is the plane of protein-based life-forms such as humans and other animals. In part, we have created it so that we can experience the challenge of being governed by emotions and instinctual desires, and the reality of being in a human body in a physical world. Here we learn how to graduate past the Fourth Plane and go forward to the Fifth Plane.

The Second Plane of Existence

This plane consists of organic material: vitamins, plants, and trees. Fairies are attracted to it because of the trees and plants.

The First Plane of Existence

This plane consists of all the inorganic material on this Earth: the minerals, crystals, soil, and rocks, all the elements that make up the Earth in its raw form, all the atoms in the periodic table before they bind to carbon bases (and so become organic).

INTERCONNECTIONS

All the planes of existence are interconnected to form the great whole of creation. Learning about the nature of each plane leads to a better understanding of these interconnections and will open us to what each plane has to teach us.

Equations

Whenever we learn to utilize the energy of one of the planes, a correspondence with another plane opens for us. This means that when we use the energy of one plane, we're using another at the same time. This is called an *equation*.

For example, the minerals from the First Plane automatically interact with the Laws of the Sixth Plane, which makes them even more effective.

Through this concept of equations we come to the realization that every plane of existence is working in our body in complete harmony to create life.

Our Connection to the Planes of Existence

We are a microcosm of the planes of existence. The human body is made up of five different compounds: lipids, carbohydrates, proteins, nucleic acid (DNA), and ATP (energy). Each of these is linked to a particular plane. Together, these five components make up who we are. They are the staff of life that connects us with the other planes.

This can be seen in the fact that our mental and spiritual health is dependent on having enough of each of these compounds. If they are lacking in our body, there will be a lack in other areas of our life as follows:

- Lack of Seventh-Plane ATP will create: *Lack of spirit and pure and unconditional love.*

- Lack of Sixth-Plane nucleic acid will create: *Lack of spiritual structure.*

- Lack of Fifth-Plane lipids will create: *Lack of spiritual balance.*

- Lack of Fourth-Plane carbohydrates will create: *Lack of energy.*

- Lack of Third-Plane proteins will create: *Lack of nurturing.*

- Lack of Second-Plane vitamins will create: *Lack of love.*

- Lack of First-Plane minerals will create: *Lack of support.*

This is why an understanding of the planes of existence is so important: *we are the seven planes of existence.*

UTILIZING THE PLANES

In the old ways, a person was expected to master the energy of one plane of existence at a time. For example, in order to know what minerals would be helpful, they would need to master the knowledge of the First Plane of Existence. Mastering the energy of a plane meant they had made a spiritual-mental shift, and this was called an initiation. This is the first time in the history of humanity that the planes of existence have been opened up simultaneously so that they can be understood and utilized as never before. In learning how to fuse the elements of the planes into a cohesive energy, we will still, however, go through lessons or initiations that will teach us how to use and understand them. Whether those lessons are hard or simple is up to us.

It is easy to become enamored by the beauty and majesty of each of the first six planes. They all have their own extraordinary belief systems, powers, and healing properties. These are brain candy, which keeps us intrigued by each plane so that we will stay there and learn all that we can.

Each plane of existence also gives us a vision of the divine filtered through it, which we interpret in our own way. I believe this is how religions are formed: a seeker makes a connection with the consciousness of a plane of existence, picks up the belief systems of that plane, and then directs them into the written word. Religious orders have been formed though the energies inherent in each plane. However, this doesn't mean that these orders haven't received information from the purity of the Seventh Plane of Existence too, since people have been touching divinity from the beginning of time.

Today, as we begin to develop our psychic abilities, we will naturally connect to the energies of the planes of existence and utilize them as the definitive self-teaching tool for spiritual growth.

2

THIS UNIVERSE ... AND BEYOND

I've always wanted to know the secrets of the universe. One day I asked the Creator, 'Where does the Seventh-Plane energy that creates particles come from?'

I was told, 'Vianna, it comes from a multi-dimensional aspect. The energy of All That Is creates this universe and the universes beyond this one, shaping all the different energies in all the different dimensions.'

The Creator started me on an exploration of the keys to bending the Laws of this universe and how they related to other dimensions. In order to understand how to bend the Laws, I first had to better comprehend our universe and how it worked three-dimensionally. This led me to have a different understanding of dimensions and how they worked.

DIMENSIONS

'Dimension' is a common term in science and metaphysics, but most people have no idea what a dimension truly is. I suggest that anyone who wishes to grasp the concept should read the book *Flatland* by Edwin Abbott. I was in third grade when my teacher read it to the class and even then it changed my life. I would miss days of school because I was sickly as a child, but when my teacher read this book to us for the first time, I really wanted to go to school. Although written more than 100 years ago in Victorian England, the book is thought-provoking, suggesting that there are answers to unknown higher realities that can be explained with scientific or rational thought if only we will free our minds to ask the right questions.

In the book, Abbott describes the life of a little square living in a two-dimensional world. He has a little house and when he meets a third-dimensional being, he is amazed that it can go into a cupboard and pull out an egg. This is a miracle to the second-dimensional square, much as it would be a miracle to us if we were to meet a fifth-dimensional being who could change from solid to spirit to solid again.

Three-Dimensional Space

Our universe is three-dimensional and this means that we are three-dimensional beings by our very nature. The Greeks conceived of three dimensions thousands of years ago using the idea of Euclidean space. Up, down, and the four cardinal directions are the three-dimensional world that we live in. This is what we are used to and how we define our universe.

We learn about three-dimensional space during infancy using what the 19th-century German physicist Hermann von Helmholtz termed *unconscious inference*, which is closely related to the development of hand and eye co-ordination. The visual ability to perceive the world in three dimensions is called *depth perception*.

As we grow older, we take for granted that three-dimensional space is the only way to perceive reality. This is one way that the body keeps us here to have an experience on this Third Plane of Existence. Because we are so strongly attached to the third dimension, the energy of another dimension would be something that we would not understand. But what if reality were more than three-dimensional space and could be defined and perceived as multi-dimensional?

I believe that there are many dimensions, each very different than our own, even into what is called the multiverse. I learned that the First, Second, and Third Planes are three-dimensional and the Fourth, Fifth, and Sixth Planes exist multi-dimensionally. They are part of this universe and a part of other dimensions as well.

As we are three-dimensional beings living on the first three planes of existence, the Fourth, Fifth, and Sixth Planes go far beyond what we imagine to be normal. We cannot even understand what fourth-dimensional energy is. We cannot conceptualize what can be done in the fourth dimension, how it differs from our three-dimensional reality, or even what it looks like. In order to understand it, we would have to experience it directly.

The way to experience these other-dimensional energies is through the spiritual consciousness of a Theta brainwave. Because spiritual thoughts travel faster than the speed of light, we can use this focused consciousness to project them past the universe we know and use them as our vehicle to experience other dimensions.

Multi-Dimensional Spirits

Although we are here on the Third Plane, our spirits are not third-dimensional in essence, but multi-dimensional. Being in a third-dimensional body seems peculiar to us when we are children, as does the rest of this third-dimensional world. As we grow older, we never quite shake the feeling that we can be and do more than this world has to offer. This is because we experienced other-dimensional energies before we came to this plane.

Everyone on this Earth is some kind of Fifth-Plane being. We are all one of two types of spiritual energy: children of the masters, and ascended masters.

Children of the Masters

Children of the masters comprise most of the soul population of Earth. They have come here from the first level of the Fifth Plane to learn and grow. They live many lifetimes, resolving the karma of negative lifetimes and working toward their mastership, learning to become beings of pure light. Once they have learned the lessons of third-dimensional energy, they are sent home to the Fifth Plane to begin an even higher phase of learning.

Ascended Masters of the Fifth Plane

The second type of spiritual energy that has come here is comprised of ascended masters from the Fifth Plane. These are spiritual beings who, over many lifetimes, have accumulated enough virtues to move up beyond this third-dimensional reality to the Fifth Plane of Existence. Completing the karma of these successive lives has brought them to a spiritual vibration high enough to become Fifth-Plane masters. If at any time they come back to this third-dimensional reality, we call them *ascended masters*. I believe that they come back to teach us the meaning of love and to help us graduate to a higher form of evolution so that we don't destroy ourselves.

Ascended masters come into this dimension with a spiritual energy that is multi-dimensional. A fully aware and awakened Fifth-Plane being can go from a solid embodiment as a human being to a spiritual embodiment. High Fifth-Plane beings are able to shift back and forth between these states *at will*.

An ascended master on this planet has the task of awakening to their full potential so that they can lead the children of the masters to enlightenment and teach them that their souls are multi-dimensional in nature.

UNDERSTANDING OUR UNIVERSE
Origins

What I was shown by the Creator was that when pure All That Is energy comes into our universe from other dimensions, it expands. Because of this, I believe that our universe is forever expanding. It is forever growing, but it isn't expanding like a balloon, because it has energy slipping in and out of it all the time. I don't believe that it is collapsing or falling apart, or that it was created by a Big Bang, but by energy seeping into an area to create atoms and to animate the Laws of the Sixth Plane. The Creator of All That Is of the Seventh Plane of Existence was the divine intelligence that caused this process to happen.

Dimensional Doorways

Then I was told that throughout the universe there were dimensional doorways of varying sizes, from very small to very large, and that these were actually what science called black holes.

I watched a show on television in 2011 that presented a theory of what was in a black hole. The idea was that when you went into a black hole you went into darkness, through layers of light into a bright golden light, through thick matter, and then into pure energy. I was struck by how similar this sounded to the process that I'd been teaching for years for going to the Seventh Plane.

I believe that there are black holes all around us, even within our own space, and when we go up in a Theta meditation, we are unconsciously directing our mind to find these dimensional doorways.

I also believe that energy gets trapped in these doorways and seeps into our third-dimensional universe from dimensions that are much more sophisticated than our own.

As I see it, black holes not only exist in certain parts of space but in every single atom as an energy field that is moving between the tiny particles in the atom. This is the energy of All That Is – the energy of creation.

Creation Energy

Creation energy consists of a pure form of love with infinite intelligence that is interconnected multi-dimensionally with all things, from the smallest particle to the largest galaxy in the universe. It is what comprises the Seventh Plane of Existence. It is everywhere – it exists in everything. It is what we utilize in a healing by connecting to the Seventh Plane. When it starts to coalesce, other energy fields are created.

The space in between creation energy is what science calls 'dark matter' but I call the Laws of the universe. Just as you have an intelligent morphogenetic field that directs DNA to perform its functions, so the multi-dimensional energy that seeps into the universe directs the Laws in much the same way.

Creation energy travels back and forth through different dimensions all the time. This is why the theory that our universe would collapse if one molecule were ever brought from another dimension into ours is ridiculous. When other-dimensional energy comes into our dimension, it takes on a new form and becomes the Law of Thought.

I believe that the other-dimensional energy that slips into our three-dimensional universe creates what quantum mechanics refers to as 'strings' in string theory. String theory is the concept that all matter is composed of vibrating filaments and membranes of energy that are multi-dimensional in nature and vibrate at specific frequencies. It is thought that these strings are the beginnings of subatomic particles. They start to move in patterns to become protons, neutrons, atoms, molecules, and finally solid matter. While this theory is not exactly the way that I believe the universe is formed, the concept of vibrating strings is similar to the way that I perceive things to be.

In my view, these tiny strings are the microcosm of this universe and the planes of existence are the macrocosm. If you go deep into the nucleus of the atom you will find protons and neutrons, and within them are particles that are even smaller, called quarks. Seventh-Plane energy coming into this universe creates the string-particles, excites them, and starts the quarks rotating to create protons and neutrons, which form the energy in the nucleus of an atom.

The number of protons in an atom make it what it is. For instance, hydrogen has one proton and one neutron, so its atomic number is one. The atomic number of gold is 79 and the atomic number of mercury is 82. (This knowledge is the key to changing the atomic structure of an element.)

The energy left over from forming the nucleus of an atom creates the small particles of energy called electrons, which revolve around the nucleus.

When I learned that the planes of existence were differentiated by how fast their atoms and molecules were vibrating, I reached an impasse of confusion about gasses, water, and solids, and how they related and worked with one another through the planes. The answer to this confusion was that the most frequent element in the universe was hydrogen.

I refer to hydrogen as the 'Father of Creation.' When oxygen starts to mix with hydrogen and carbon, the 'Mother of Creation,' we have what we perceive as life.

Two hydrogen atoms and one oxygen atom form water, which can be a gas (steam), a solid (ice), and a liquid (water). So, in its different forms, it has the energy to take our consciousness between the different planes of existence. It is the bridge between the planes.

This explains why some people have spiritual experiences in or around water. In fact, the meditation that I use to teach the journey to the Seventh Plane was taught to me while I was in a steaming hot tub of water.

In this meditation, we are sending the energy of our consciousness through the vast expanses of the universe, riding on a timeless Theta wave that travels many times the speed of light through the Laws into the pearlescent light of Seventh-Plane energy. While we are in this energy, we can become it in order to witness using it to create a healing. This is how to do it:

GO UP TO THE SEVENTH PLANE OF EXISTENCE!

Ground and center yourself.

Begin by sending your consciousness down into the center of Mother Earth, which is a part of All That Is. Bring the energy up through your feet, into your body and up through all the chakras.

Go up through your crown chakra in a beautiful ball of light. Imagine that ball of light going out past the stars and through the universe.

Go beyond the universe, past the layers of light, through a golden light, past the jelly-like substance that is the Laws, past a deep blue light, past a pink mist and into a pearlescent white light, the Seventh Plane of Existence, the pure energy of creation. This is the energy that creates the particles that create atoms.

In this meditation, the golden light is the Christ energy of unconditional love. The reason why you go past the deep blue light, which is the Law of Magnetism, is to avoid getting distracted by it. It will talk to you and you will have a lovely time, but you can commune with it for hours. If you wish, talk to it after you have gone to the Seventh Plane.

The luminescent snow-white light of the Seventh Plane will seem formless, but it sparkles with energy and may have a few sparkles of pink and blue in it. This means it is suffused with the combined energies of truth and compassion. This is the highest truth. As you contact this energy of creation, you will see that it is pouring into our third-dimensional universe from the Fourth, Fifth, Sixth, and Seventh Planes and forming atoms. You are reaching this pure energy before it becomes an atom. You can then direct it, by the power of thought, into someone's space to 'dis-create' sickness and create life.

I always knew that I was going to a place of pure love and pure energy to perform a healing. I was not only 'going up', but also 'expanding out' into the energy. As you expand with pure thought, you learn to pull the pure energy of love to you in its highest form.

The following exercise enables you to bring this All That Is energy into your own space.

EXPANDING INTO THE SEVENTH PLANE OF EXISTENCE

Seat yourself in a comfortable chair or on a sofa and take a deep breath in.

Imagine that you and the chair have become one on a molecular level. Your molecules and those of the chair are transferring back and forth between one another. You are connecting to the molecules, becoming one with them.

Now imagine that on a molecular level you are a part of everything in the room. Expand and become one with the outside world.

Imagine that you are a part of the area, then the country that you are in.

Imagine that you are a part of the entire Earth, connecting to earth, land, and sea, every creature, every nation on this planet until you and the Earth are one.

Imagine that you and the universe are one.

Imagine that you are a part of all the bright white and golden lights.

Imagine that you are a part of the jelly-like substance.

Finally, imagine that you are a part of the iridescent white light that is the Seventh Plane of Existence. Become one with this iridescent white light.

Think to yourself, *Creator of All That Is, thank you for my life.*

Take a deep breath in and open your eyes.

Welcome to the Seventh Plane of Existence. Behold, you are not separate, you are a part of God, of All That Is.

I believe that when we go up to the Seventh Plane, we're taking them within their own brain to the message-carriers, the neurons. We go within the very energy that connects the neural pathways to the cells. By doing this, we become aware that they are connected to every molecule, to every atom, to all the energy associated with subatomic particles...

The massive power of the universe is within us and all around us, waiting for us to find it through the energy of pure thought. Once this power has been recognized within, it will flow outward, expanding through the planes of existence into the immense macrocosm of the Creator of All That Is. It will be this inner awareness that will bring us to the realization that we no longer have the need for the incredible competition that there is among us today, and the battle of duality will be over.

THOUGHTS – FASTER THAN LIGHT SPEED

With our present technology, we can build all kinds of machines, and the last frontier is the exploration of consciousness and the power of our thoughts. Think of the endless possibilities if we were able to move matter with the power of our thoughts! It would be possible to change an atom of mercury to an atom of gold with the energy of a thought, just as the ancient alchemists attempted to do. But by the time we reach this level of attainment, gold won't have any more value than mercury, so why do it in the first place? The thing that will have real value will be the ability to heal. Gold will only have value for its intrinsic vibrations, not for its monetary worth.

So, what is really happening with the process that we call a thought? What is it exactly? Can it be defined using our limited third-dimensional concepts?

Obviously, thoughts are a type of energy unto themselves and can influence matter, since we use them to move our body. But what if we could do more with them? What if we were able to project them in a way that defied current scientific explanation? What if there are energies that modern physics has not yet discovered?

In this universe, I believe there are different forms of energy that can shift protons and atoms around, most of which are under the Laws of the Sixth Plane. One of these energies is pure thought.

Some of these forms of energy have been discovered, while others have yet to be explored. The following are some that have been discovered:

- electricity

- magnetism

- velocity/combustion

- atomic energy (uranium plutonium)

- hydrogen

- biological energy

- chemical reactions

- light-heat

- sound-vibration

These are others that have yet to be fully explored:

- pyramid energy

- lestosive energy – use of electrons

- quark movement/string theory

- sacred geometry

- dimensional energy

- pure thought

Pure thought is one of the energies that we are exploring in this book. I believe that it is possible to move matter by pure thought – if you know how. The universe was created by the unbelievable energy of the pure thought-form of *love*, which is now seeping into our world as pure energy. The understanding of this thought-energy will permit us to become inter-dimensional beings. The first time that you are pure of thought, things such as teleportation can spontaneously happen. Thoughts can move between dimensions, but only if they have a high vibration – thoughts of love, gratitude, and compassion, for example. Low-vibrational thoughts, such as thoughts of hatred, malevolence, and greed, keep us trapped in the prison of the third dimension. The way to move beyond this dimension is with a 'lite' thought-form.

The Lite Thought-form

I believe that what I call a 'lite thought-form' is the purest and most powerful form of energy in this universe. I refer to it as 'lite' instead of 'light' because even light has enough weight to be heavier than a lite thought-form. This is 'lite' because it must work similarly to the energy of light while being able to travel faster than the speed of light. It cannot be heavy, as that will anchor it to the Earth. If it is lite, it can leave the confines of the Earth ... and this dimension.

What are 'heavy' thoughts? They are ones that never get off the planet, anchors that keep us in a familiar paradigm on Earth, which is one reason why we are so attached to creating them. Fear, doubt, disbelief, hatred, and resentment are just some of them.

Be careful not to create negative thoughts that will anchor you to this Third-Plane illusion!

I believe that there was a time when we communicated using thoughts instead of words, but as we developed verbal communication we forgot how. As a consequence, we've also forgotten how to control our negative thoughts.

But our thoughts and our spirit are what direct our life. Our thoughts and emotions make us what we are. In order for the spiritual essence that is in our Third-Plane body to perform healings, our thoughts must be as pure as possible. If we attempt to do a healing when we have a heavy thought, it isn't going to happen.

So, if you're doing a healing and a heavy thought-form goes through your mind, stop and wait until you're projecting a lite thought-form before starting again. You only have to keep your thoughts pure for two or three minutes in order to do a healing or body scan, or to read someone's thoughts.

Thought-forms are very powerful. The right kind of lite thought-form can bend the Laws of the universe. These lite thought-forms are called virtues. (We'll look at these in more detail later.)

EXPRESSIONS OF POWER

As our Fifth-Plane soul integrates with this Third-Plane illusion, the ability to manifest with the power of the spoken word, the focused thought, and even the strong emotion will expand expeditiously.

The things we say and the strong thought-forms we have are magnified by the use of Theta waves. This is because when we're in Theta we connect not only to our own divinity but directly to the divine, to the pure essence of the Seventh Plane. Because this is creation energy, it's important to be aware of any random thoughts or expressions and the way that we project them. There's an emotional component attached to words and thought-forms that doesn't always proceed in a logical manner. So we not only have to watch what we say and think, but also find out *why* we're saying or thinking it.

Think about all the words and thought-forms that are in your paradigm. What do they mean to you on all levels of your being? Perhaps they're blocking you from progressing without you knowing it. As you develop your intuitive abilities, your words, thought-forms, and belief systems will all have the power to create changes in your daily life, for good or ill. If a statement is voiced enough times, it will become 'reality.' If a thought is formed in a deep enough Theta brainwave, instant manifestation is possible.

Once you're able to manifest changes with the power of thought, you must particularly watch what you say and think. If you have a negative thought or make a negative statement, always say, 'Cancel.'

Deep belief work may be needed to distinguish between fears that can cause manifestations and fears that do not. Not every thought or statement is going to bring about a manifestation, but it's very important to be aware of what you might be creating. (*For belief work, see page 41 and the appendix.*)

When you connect to the Creator and bring the All That Is energy into a reading, it's important to listen to the 'words' of the Creator. If you permit your fears, doubts, or lack of belief to enter into the reading, your communication with the Creator will be filtered through your belief systems.

It is awareness of how thought-forms and the spoken word have the power to develop a *living consciousness* that is important. By exploring your psyche and the psyche of your clients with belief work, you can learn if a spoken word or subconscious program is creating dysfunction.

We all know how powerful words can be. Gossip and thoughtless words can cause emotional pain. As a process of personal growth, many people learn not to say what they think. If we could read one another's minds consistently, we'd *really* get our feelings hurt!

Whether we're aware of it or not, we actually sense and filter other people's thoughts all the time. There are times when we're bombarded with negative thoughts from people who enjoy not liking us. When you feel these vibrations, you can allow them to affect you or not – it's your choice. There are going to be some people who don't like you or what you do. But if you permit others to like and respect you, this will change. You have to be ready to receive love back from people and not to expect dislike. One way to avoid it is to cultivate forgiveness and live your life connected to the consciousness of the Seventh Plane of Existence. (*For a forgiveness exercise, see page 35.*)

THE SEVENTH PLANE OF EXISTENCE: ALL THAT IS

After thousands of consultations with clients, I began to notice that many intuitive individuals were focused on the energy inherent in one particular plane of existence at a time. I found that because of this they were bound by the rules of that plane and became attached to it to the exclusion of all others.

I started to realize that there had to be a single all-encompassing energy that brought all the planes of existence together. Then, through an initiation from the planes of existence, I learned how to go to the Seventh Plane by going beyond the Laws themselves. This was when I was able to find the road map to the Creator of All That Is.

From the moment that I went to the Seventh Plane, I realized that I'd never been separate from the Creator of All That Is. There is no separation other than the illusion we create to keep ourselves here on the Third Plane. We are always part of All That Is.

Seventh-Plane Principles

The Seventh Plane of Existence is the pure energy of All That Is. It is all-encompassing. Unlike the energy of the other six planes, it simply embraces us in love while changing our human vibration to perfection.

When we become aware that we can use the All That Is energy that is the Seventh Plane easily and effortlessly, we can create our reality. With this awareness, time ceases to exist. All separation based upon duality disappears, to reveal the pure essence of the divine and loving Creator of All That Is.

Through the Creator, instant healings, instant accountability, and instant results are created. Problems aren't fixed, just changed, because another reality is created – with a thought. Thought is the one tangible energy that is fast enough to influence the energy of a proton and neutron. So, as a healer sends a lite thought-form to the Seventh Plane, it connects to the energy of All That Is, and the healer takes with them an image of the present reality and witnesses it being replaced by an image of what the reality should be.

To heal sickness, I tell students to reach into the atomic energy of All That Is and imagine that we are all made of atoms, then take the pattern of sickness and witness it being replaced with the pattern of health. This realigns those atoms in the proper way. No matter what the sickness is, you can literally move it into the energy of All That Is and bring out health and wholeness.

From this microcosmic standpoint, we understand the Seventh Plane as the energy that creates the very particles that make up atoms. It is the subatomic source of All That Is. It is creation itself, the fountainhead of all life and more.

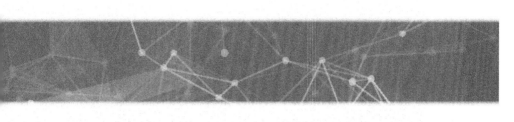

3

THE LAWS OF THE SIXTH PLANE: VIRTUES OF ASCENSION

The universe is held together by the incredible energy of the Laws. These are condensed thought-forms with a high frequency of vibration that can take on forms as group consciousness to communicate with us. They have such a high energy that they are able to transcend the First, Second, Third, Fourth, and Fifth-Plane energies to become the universal bond that holds everything together. Not only do they hold together this universe, but multi-dimensional universes as well.

The Sixth Plane of Existence is composed of the essence of the Laws. The Sixth Plane has been called the great void (or dark matter), which is part of the jelly-like substance that we travel through to get to the Seventh Plane in my meditation.

There are Laws that govern our universe, our galaxy, our solar system, the Earth, and even us. There are Laws that govern the Fifth, Fourth, Third, Second, and First Planes of Existence. These Laws create an imaginary division between the different planes, but they truly all exist together. They are the Laws of physics: the Law of Magnetism, the Law of Electricity, the Law of Truth, the Law of Nature, the Law of Compassion, the Law of Gravity, the Law of Time, and many others.

The Laws of the universe are a giant group consciousness of their own. They give us the realization that we are having a life experience. They create the structure for the reality that we exist, that we breathe, and that we are human.

We are fortunate to be able to use some of the Laws at will. For instance, we use electricity every day when we flip a light switch.

As Third-Plane beings from the Fifth Plane of Existence, we can get information directly from a Law, and we can also learn to bend space using thought and create machines and atomic energy. Throughout history, people have been born who have received information from Laws and, as a result, have helped the vibration of humankind ascend. People such as Plato, Aristotle, Leonardo da Vinci, Galileo, Newton, Tesla, Edison, and Einstein were all born with the ability to channel information from the Laws. For instance, Tesla channeled the Law of Magnetism and the Law of Electricity. When Galileo proposed that the Earth was round, his ideas were not very popular and many people made fun of him. The Church told him that he had better change his mind, because the Earth was flat. But he was sure that it was round. This inspiration came from the intelligence of the Laws.

Healers who use the Laws of the Sixth Plane of Existence will do healings with tones, colors, sacred geometry or geometric shapes, numbers or numerology, magnetism or the Earth's magnetic grid, astrology or light. Sometimes, when you do healings, the Creator will send you to the Sixth Plane of Existence, where you may hear tones, see colors, and get mathematical formulas for illnesses. It is the Laws that teach the mathematics of an atom.

The philosophy on the Sixth Plane is: 'If it's broken, fix it.' Often healers here get caught up in overelaborate explanations that require enormous amounts of energy. Healers who use the Laws often become blunt in their truth and are easily irritated at themselves and others in their quest for 'Truth.' To hold this and other types of 'Law vibration' for long periods of time is hard on the human body. It takes a great deal of persistence and practice to hold these kinds of energy, but if love is used it can be done. The Sixth Plane has a strong vibration that imposes truth and accountability on the person that connects to it.

It is important for those who use the Sixth Plane of Existence to come to the realization that they are living in an illusion and directing their own illusion. They know they no longer need to punish themselves in order to grow and progress. On this plane, the battle between good and evil is eliminated and replaced by pure Truth. People who work exclusively on this plane are sometimes called *mystics*.

Each Law is a huge consciousness that has smaller ones connected to it. It has a spirit-like essence, a living, moving consciousness. You should never permit or ask for the complete essence of a Law to come into your space or into your body, as this can cause problems that are best avoided. The human body is too fragile. You should connect with the Seventh Plane of Existence prior to speaking with the Laws outside your physical 'space.'

You can invite a Law to speak with you, but it is up to the Law whether and when it accepts the invitation. You can speak with these beings through the Seventh Plane of Existence, but to work with them you have to master virtues. Virtues are positive moral characteristics that guide the way we live our lives. They steer the ship of our spirit to the Laws.

PRINCIPLES OF THE LAWS

The Laws of the universe are the structure of the Sixth Plane of Existence. They are always at work around us and interact with us daily. Good examples of Laws that are working for us every day are the Laws of Gravity and Time, Magnetism, and Electricity.

One of the Laws that you will connect to when doing Theta work is the Law of Truth, which will help you throughout your life. The Law of Compassion is often at the doorway of the Seventh Plane of Existence. It appears pink and cloud-like. As the saying goes, 'It is through compassion that you reach the Creator of All That Is.'

Laws can be bent, such as when an airplane takes flight and velocity outweighs gravity. You can bend the Law of Electricity by flipping a light switch. The next step would be to let the electricity flow out of your fingertips.

There is a big difference between bending Laws and using Laws on this Third Plane of Existence. We use Laws all the time. The combustion engine is another good example of this. We drive down the road at 70 miles per hour, but we may not understand the inner workings of this Law – we simply use it. But the people who first built the combustion engine had to understand and channel the Law in order to build the engine in the first place. There was a time when people believed that if you traveled faster than 60 miles per hour, you would fly apart! But there was someone who thought otherwise, and look at us now!

Tesla had to understand certain Laws in order to implement the Laws of Electricity and Magnetism in this reality. He could have been born with a genetic predisposition to certain virtues and that may have given him genetic tendencies to connect to the different energies of certain Laws. Men like this have always been at the forefront of invention.

Harmonious Laws

We all are born with a Law that is special to us. For instance, I am fascinated by the Law of Truth and I think that this Law is part of my quest. I think that many people who realize that they are sparks of God will evolve enough to be closely connected to and in harmony with a particular Law. I think that many of us will develop an affinity to a Law of the universe once we begin to realize this connection.

The Laws have been some of my best teachers, and from my experience with them, they are beyond emotional outbursts. Some people say that they can channel the Laws, but people experiencing great emotional eruptions are not channeling the Laws, because the Laws are essentially beyond negative emotions.

It is possible to learn a great deal from the Laws. After a teaching from them, you will feel supercharged.

The Major Laws

Here is a small list of major Laws. It is not a complete list – there are actually millions of Laws – but these Laws are the ones we are expected to know in this lifetime.

- Under the Law of Truth come the Law of Prophecy and the Law of Motion, which states, 'Once in motion, always in motion.' Under the Law of Motion are the Law of Free Agency and the Law of Thought: 'I think, therefore I am.' Also under the Law of Motion come the Law of Velocity and the Law of Cause and Effect (sometimes called the

Law of Karma). Under the Law of Cause and Effect are the Law of Wisdom, the Law of Action, and the Law of Justice. Under the Law of Justice is the Law of Witness or Acceptance. The Law of Witness is the very powerful rule that something has to be witnessed before it can happen.

- Under the Law of Magnetism is the Law of Gravity. Under the Law of Gravity are the Law of Time and the Law of Attraction. Under the Law of Time are the Law of Sacred Geometry and the Law of Dimensions. (Avoid getting caught up in the Law of Dimensions, as there are many dimensions.) Under the Law of Dimensions is the Law of Illusion, which keeps you thinking that you're here. Under the Law of Illusion is the Law of DNA, which is connected to all DNA. The Akashic Records or the Hall of Records are also under the Law of Time.

- Under the Law of Vibration is the Law of Energy, and under the Law of Energy is the Law of Focus. Under the Law of Focus are the Law of Light, the Law of Tones, and the Law of Electricity.

- The Law of Compassion has the ability to bend many Laws. Under the Law of Compassion are the Law of Pure Intent, the Law of Patience, and the Law of Emotion. (There is no Law of Love. Love is a pure Seventh Plane of Existence Energy. *It just is* and is supreme.)

- The Law of Nature has a name, and her name is Oma. The Law of Nature rules everything that has to do with the Earth and this galaxy. There are Laws under her, such as the Law of Balance. The Law of Nature is always changing and improving upon the Law of Life. Under the Law of Life are the elements – earth, water, fire, and air. There is no Law of the Creation of Life, because the true energy of creation is the All That Is energy of the Seventh Plane of Existence of pure love.

There are many more Laws than those mentioned here.

MEET WITH A LAW

In order to meet with a Law, you have to go up above your space to the Seventh Plane (*see pages 13 and 14*) and ask the Creator of All That Is to introduce you to a Law. You must *invite* a Law to come to you. You may meet with the Law of Cause and Effect, which sometimes shows itself as two mirrors or as two waterfalls. Or perhaps you will meet the Law of Compassion, which presents itself as pink fluffy clouds. Sometimes the Laws present themselves as large faces and balls of energy.

Invite a Law to come to you and introduce itself and you will have an experience. Do not be surprised if you have it again consciously over the next few days with your eyes and ears, because Laws can take physical form in order to communicate with you.

Always go to the Creator first before doing any other work. And remember to stay focused. Otherwise, you could get lost in the brain candy of the Sixth Plane.

You are only being introduced to a Law here. You cannot bend a Law until you have mastered virtues.

Welcome to the world of the Laws.

1. Go up to the Seventh Plane of Existence (*see pages 13 and 14*) and invite a Law to come to you by saying: '*Creator of All That Is, it is requested to connect with a Law of the Sixth Plane of Existence. Thank you. It is done, it is done, it is done.*'

2. Witness meeting a Law through the Creator of All That Is.

3. When you choose to return, move your consciousness out of the Sixth Plane of Existence, rinse yourself off with Seventh-Plane energy and stay connected to it.

It is easiest to meet with your harmonious Law, a Law that has been connected to you from the beginning.

MEET WITH YOUR HARMONIOUS LAW

1. Go up to the Seventh Plane and invite the Law to come to you by saying: *'Creator of All That Is, I ask to know the Sixth-Plane Law with which I am in harmony. Show me in the highest and best way.'*

2. Meet with the Law and get to know it.

3. When you have finished, rinse yourself off with Seventh-Plane energy and stay connected to it.

Physical Laws and Emotional Laws

Essentially, there are two different kinds of Law in the universe: physical Laws and emotional Laws. Sometimes an emotion or a virtue is so powerful it becomes a Law. For instance, the Law of Compassion can bend physical Laws like the Laws of Electricity and Magnetism, yet it is an *emotional* Law.

How the Laws Work

Some Laws can be bent, while others can be broken. One of the very first Laws that can be bent is the Law of Time. Many ThetaHealers can bend the Law of Time because they have the basic attributes (virtues) needed for this talent, such as compassion and wanting to help the planet. These basic attributes make it easy to bend this Law.

You just *bend* the Law of Time, you don't *break* it. You don't stop time for the whole planet, you only affect your own paradigm, your own microcosmic world. I don't slow down the rotation of the Earth simply because I want to. That would utilize a different Law, one that I am not able to bend: an Ultimate Truth.

Laws that we cannot change are called *Ultimate Truths*. The Law of the Rotation of the Planes and the Law of Free Agency are Ultimate Truths. The Law of Free Agency means that you have free agency and are sharing this planet with billions of other souls who also have free agency. Laws that are Ultimate Truths supersede *lesser* Laws.

To interact with a Law, *you must first go to the Seventh Plane*. In order to connect to the pure essence of a Law, you must filter it through the Seventh Plane of Existence.

If you want to anchor the energy of the Law or to use and apply that energy, you must possess the virtues to connect with it (*see below*). Then you must ask for the name of the Law. The name of the Law is a tone or vibration that you have to use to interact with it. Then you wait for the energy, vibration, and information to come into you.

VIRTUES AND VICES

Virtues are thought-patterns that move faster than the speed of light. They can bend time and space. When you master a virtue, you are also mastering a high-vibrational thought-form. Once your thoughts are of a high enough vibration, they can connect to a Law and work in unison with it. But negative thoughts and the vices that are attached to them never leave the Earth's magnetic pull. Nothing else shows the fundamental truth of the duality of the Third Plane of Existence better than virtues and vices.

Most virtues come with learning experiences that include vices, or negative thoughts to overcome in order to attain the virtues. Eradication of vices goes hand in hand with cultivating virtues.

We use vices as motivation to go forward. They are not our enemy; on the contrary, they are designed to make us feel safe and secure. They create a 'comfort zone' for us. For instance, if we have resentment and hatred for an abusive parent, it keeps that person away. It keeps a barrier between us and the person. Our subconscious is trying to keep us protected. It keeps us feeling resentment too, but often resentment is also connected to positive lessons.

One of the reasons why some people do not master virtues is because of their attachment to this plane and the relationships that they have with family and friends. They are afraid that if they progress too far spiritually, they may move beyond the third dimension and leave their friends and family behind. You have no idea how much your spirit loves your family and friends in this existence.

On an intrinsic level, however, the soul already knows that it must develop virtues. It creates situations so that we can develop the virtues for whatever goal it is seeking to attain. So, things that seem wrong in our life are not amiss on a higher level. We create every negative (or positive) situation in order to raise our level of vibration. It is how we react to these situations that dictates the depth of pain and misery, or joy and happiness, that we experience in our daily life.

Our challenge is to live in a state of pure love, unaffected by all the negativity in this existence. One way to do this is to find out what we are creating in our life. It is true that our soul is always creating something for us to learn. But when we focus our thoughts, we can be aware of what it is creating.

If the Creator wants me to learn how to be kind, for instance, then I can go out and be kind to 10 people a day and learn kindness that way instead of learning through difficult situations. In this way we can focus on what we are supposed to do, and that should be our divine timing. Our divine timing is the reason we are here – our mission in this life.

Your soul already knows much of what I am teaching you. It knows what virtue it came to learn as part of its divine timing. Even an ascended master who has come to this Earth as a tutor is open to learning extra virtues.

What is important is to be able to implement virtues at will.

Bending the Laws by Acquiring Virtues

As important as it is to have virtues, it is also important to be able to direct our thoughts and send them with kindness, love, harmony, and humility. These energies are created by having enough virtues to influence a Law. For instance, inter-dimensional beings on the Fourth and Fifth Planes of Existence exist with us on this plane and outside our dimension at the same time, and have the ability to shift between dimensions at will. The way that they develop this ability is by mastering virtues to access and bend the Laws. Once you reach the right vibrational level to manipulate a Law, that Law will begin to interact with you and give you information.

The Laws are the weave of the fabric of the universe. There is a way to bend almost any Law of the universe, and thought is the way to do it. But the thought must be pure – a lite thought – and precisely directed into the atomic structure of the beginning of all creation.

In order to understand how to bend certain Laws of this universe with your thoughts, you must have the sacred name of the Law and a thought process that has a vibration high enough to reach the thought-form of the Law in question – that is to say, you must have the right virtue.

Most of the holy books, including the Holy Bible, the Torah, the Buddhist *Dhammapada*, the *Bhagavad Gita* and the Koran, talk about embracing virtues to push out negative emotion and avoid negative acts. The ancients understood the importance of avoiding negative thoughts. Both ancient and more modern scriptures teach us about the power of pure thought and the importance of virtues. All of the scriptures tell us to keep evil thoughts, such as jealousy, hatred, greed, and resentment, away from us. Wise men and women of ancient times did not directly understand molecules of emotion as we do now, but they still understood on an instinctual level that negative feelings created problems in their lives.

So we have been offered guidance on virtues many times in the past; however, because of our limitations, we have only been able to accept this message in fragments. It takes a great deal of spiritual courage to accept this knowledge, and in earlier times neither the ruling class nor the majority of the population had the capacity for this kind of commitment to virtue. In the present day, this is changing.

While it is important to develop virtues, you have to be able to apply and fuse them together in the right way. You may only need a little of one kind of virtue but the energy of many others to manipulate a Law. ThetaHealers do this all the time. They go up to the Creator and visualize a healing using not only the virtue of faith, but also those of restraint, kindness, forgiveness, gratitude, acceptance, wonder, hope, service, courage, and compassion. These blends are needed to do healings consistently and to activate each Law. They allow us to raise our vibration to a level on which we can understand the Laws, connect with them, and bend them in a pure way. It is our birthright to realize our connection to All That Is, but virtues give us the desire to do this by holding a pure frequency of vibration.

If you only have three of the blends of virtues out of the five that are required to work through a Law, it may not be possible to let God do the work of an instant healing. If you are missing a certain virtue and your soul decides to connect to the Law of Truth, then things will automatically come up in your life to make it possible for you to acquire that virtue. So, challenges will start coming into your life.

Mastering Virtues

How do you know when you have learned enough to have mastered a virtue? By acknowledging that you have mastered it, practicing it, and feeling the change within you. You *will* feel the change, especially when you realize what the universe is trying to teach you. Life is not designed to torture you, but to teach you.

This is part of the awakening. The awakening is the realization that you are a Fifth-Plane being living in this illusion who wants to progress through the levels of the Fifth Plane.

The more virtues you acquire, the easier it is to work with people and understand them. The more healings you do, the more people you reach. The more people you reach, the more people you change. The more people you change, the higher your frequency becomes on this plane in preparation for the next evolution.

In this way, progressing to a new level of evolution is made possible by acquiring virtues. Mastering a virtue changes the frequency of a thought-form so it can connect with a particular Law. Certain virtues connect to certain Laws and so it becomes possible to work through those Laws at all times.

THE VIRTUES OF THE LAWS

The following are some of the virtues required to bend the Laws: acceptance, assertiveness, authenticity, beauty, belief, bravery, caring, charisma, clarity, cleanliness, cleverness, commitment, communication, compassion, confidence, consideration, contentment, conviction, cooperation, courage, creativity, curiosity, dedication, detachment, determination, devotion, dignity, endurance, enjoyment, enthusiasm, excellence, fairness, faith, flexibility, focus, forgiveness, fortitude, friendliness, generosity, gentleness, grace, graciousness, gratitude, harmony, helpfulness, honesty, honor, hope, humility, humor, idealism, imagination, integrity, intelligence, joyfulness, justice, kindness, love, loyalty, mercy, moderation, modesty, morality, nobility, optimism, orderliness, passion, patience, peace, perseverance, playfulness, preparedness, pure intent, purposefulness, reliability, respect, responsibility, reverence, self-discipline, service, sincerity, sympathy, tact, temperance, tenaciousness, thankfulness, tolerance, trust, truthfulness, understanding, unity, vision, wisdom, and wonder.

The following paragraphs give examples of virtues and vices as a means of explaining how these thought-forms benefit and hinder us.

The Virtue of Service

When I first started to do healings I became obsessed with the energy of an instant healing. When an instant healing happens for the first time you feel happy and feel love for the world, at least for an hour or two until something grounds you. When you experience the energy of an instant healing in more and more people, the feeling of happiness and love lasts longer. In some instances, one person will receive an instant healing and several other people will receive an instant healing directly after that. When this happens, you will walk around in joy for two or three days and it becomes unnecessary to sleep and eat.

When this first happened to me, there was a side effect: when the euphoria wore off, I became depressed, sad and grumpy. Because of these ups and downs during my day, when I finally got off work I would have to take a bath to wash off my day before I could talk to anybody. Then I learned to stay connected to the energy of All That Is so that I didn't have these mood swings. I trained my mind to know that I was always connected to it.

This energy is not connected to me; I am connected to it. It doesn't start with me, because we are all connected to All That Is. I don't control the whole world, but I am part of it. So I can move this energy and create what I need to so that I can progress.

I found that if I made the extra effort and put the needs of others before my own and took a little extra time with people who were sick, I could hold that energy for longer. The lesson I learned was the virtue of *service*.

The Virtue of Tolerance

It is very important to develop tolerance in order to understand who we are and to understand others. Being able to tolerate the world around us enables us to see it clearly. If we don't have true tolerance, we can't see the full truth. If someone comes to us for healing and we see only the good and not the bad, we will push the truth away because we don't have the tolerance to see it. If we want to see inside someone else's heart, we have to be able to see truth, and this takes tolerance. In order to see into the future, we have to have true tolerance for humankind. One of the reasons why many people are not good healers is because they dislike their own kind – other humans – not to mention their human body. Tolerance is being able to let things be as they are, being largely unaffected by them, and moving forward.

One of the reasons that I can see into my students' lives is because I know that I have the ability to love them and to accept what they do in their lives, even if I do not agree with everything that they do. I know my intention to help them is pure, because I don't insert my own opinion and because I do my best to let the Creator of All That Is talk through me.

If you are having strange stressful situations with the people in your life, it may be that you are being taught tolerance.

The Virtue of Courage

*Courage is not the absence of fear, but rather the judgment
that something else is more important than fear.*
You may not live forever, but the over-cautious may not live at all.

Courage is when we face our fears and follow through. Sometimes we think that we are fighting evil, but it is our own inner fears that are against us. But even fighting our fears and negative habits shows us that we can accomplish things, even when it seems that the odds are not in our favor. This is why it is important to master the virtue of courage.

Courage is one of the virtues that bind many other virtues together, because without courage, many of them would not exist. They would fall apart, because it takes courage to learn a virtue. We should have the courage to say, 'Let's see if this works,' the courage to say, 'I'm praying to the Creator,' and the courage to say, 'I believe in the Creator of All That Is,' or at least, 'I believe.'

If your healings are only working part of the time, then you may have a lower-grade thought-form in your brain that is blocking you. It takes courage to have an awareness of these dysfunctional thought-forms and even more courage to clean them out so that healing can happen.

The Virtue of Bravery

Bravery has a different energy than courage. It is the absence of fear. It is something that we just have. It is also a magnificent virtue.

Both bravery and courage are required in life. Bravery is often developed after courage.

The Virtue of Forgiveness

You cannot 'fake it until you make it' with virtues such as, for example, joy. Being joyful is a virtue that must be learned on a soul level. The only thing that you can 'fake until you make it' is the virtue of forgiveness. This can be done by repeating the pure thought *I forgive you, I forgive you, I forgive you* over and over again until eventually you develop the virtue of pure forgiveness.

Forgiveness has such a high vibration that just saying the word can protect you. Forgiving others can dissolve negative energy and thoughts as well as reflect them back to the sender.

In the Bible it says to forgive your enemies. This gives you protection from them. Forgiveness is the highest protection there is.

PROTECTION THROUGH FORGIVENESS

Most of us can think of someone who dislikes or even hates us. Please don't misunderstand me – most of your 'enemies' are not worth your time, but I want you to think of someone who is sending you negative thoughts, or someone who has done wrong to you in your life. You should imagine doing this exercise with only one person at a time.

1. Go up and connect to the Creator (*see pages 13 and 14*) and imagine that the person who has hurt you is standing in front of you.

2. Imagine telling this person how they have hurt you and what they have done to you.

3. Imagine telling the person that you forgive them for hurting you. As you do so, watch their reaction.

   If they are still standing in front of you in the vision and they say that they are sorry, it means that they feel remorse for what they have done. If you come to the realization that they feel remorse, then the energy of forgiveness will protect you from any angry thought-forms that they send you. This will also allow you to have compassion for them.

   If they disappear into ash in the vision, this means that they have no remorse and this takes away all negative thoughts from you. The hateful person will have to deal with their own negative thoughts and they can no longer affect you. This means that what you have to learn from this person is done and you are protected from them.

   If they are still standing in front of you in the vision without saying anything, what you have to learn from them is not finished. This means that you have to do belief work on the situation. As you free yourself from the obligation of what they have to teach you, they will begin to get smaller and smaller in the vision.

   In some instances the person will apologize to you and it may be that they can make amends.

In any event, forgiveness is the strongest protection because when you say 'I forgive you' to someone, this means that you are no longer accepting any negative energy from them.

The Vice of Criticalness

One of the easiest vices to fall into is being critical of ourself and others. As long as we are over-critical, we cannot step out of our comfort zone and achieve full enlightenment. When we practice ThetaHealing, we have to be able to get rid of (or at least control) our critical tendencies, at least for the time that we are healing.

Humans are interesting creatures. Because of survival reflexes, we have compared ourselves to other humans for so long that it has become a collective subconscious program. It has become instinctual. We constantly compare our intelligence, our health, and our body to those of other people. We compare our clothing, jewelry, and even how much money we make.

To get out of this habit and other types of heavy thinking may take some practice. However, once this becomes your conscious goal, the Creator will give you plenty of people to practice on. You will meet people who are reflections of your heavy thought-forms until you have mastered this virtue.

Criticalness is one of the heavy thought-forms that will quickly lower your vibration. This will block you from moving forward. There are many people on the Earth who don't want to move forward and it is ultimately up to each of us to decide for ourselves. But this is the only time in history that we have been able to acquire all the virtues in one lifetime instead of only learning one or two virtues each life.

Why are we allowed to achieve all the virtues in this lifetime? Because we already have them! They are already ours. We just have to remember them in this Third-Plane body. We have the opportunity to integrate our spiritual self with our physical self and become aware of the virtues we already have. How else could we teach love to the masters of the children?

For every person we awaken, every person we give hope and love to, every person we make a difference to, we advance on a soul level. Some of us want to advance to the higher soul levels so that we can help not just a few people but millions of people. Some of us will write books to wake up millions. Some of will us teach classes to wake up millions. It is not likely that most of us will be satisfied with waking up just one person, but we should remember that one individual might in turn wake up millions. In any case, we came here with the obligation to wake others and what we can achieve is limitless.

The Vice of Egotism

One of the vices that always stops us from developing virtues is egotism, or being egotistical. This brings forth karma. I have witnessed this among many of my clients and students. Competition to be the 'best healer' is a perfect example of egotism. Remember, *the best healer is the Creator of All That Is and our job is to witness the healings.*

To take another instance, there have been many people in my classes who have said that they can tell me what I am thinking. Generally, what they tell me I am thinking is completely wrong. What they are telling me is what is in *their* mind. Their egotism isn't allowing them to see the truth.

There is a difference between being egotistical and acknowledging that you have a gift. Egotism can block you from using many skills. If you are too egotistical, you will block yourself from becoming who you really are and learning what you need to work on. Do you really have certain attributes or do you just *think* you do? It may be that you are ahead of yourself spiritually and your ego is naturally keeping people away from you.

An ego is not a bad thing. A healthy ego defines how we dress, how we move; it's what defines us. But egotism is when we think, *It's all about me,* and it can border on narcissism. An egotistical person thinks that everyone exists for them. It is important to know the difference between the ego and being egotistical. This keeps our ego in check and avoids the problems egotism can cause.

A good way to keep the ego balanced is to have the capacity to love others as *they* need to be loved. This may make us a little vulnerable. But many of us made a promise to wake people up before we came here, which means we have to take a chance in helping them.

When we are witnessing God doing healings, we may have some successes in healings and readings. This is why we always give credit to God the Creator. God is the healer. We are the witness. If a healer gets confused about this, the universe has a way of clarifying it for them. I sometimes see this in students new to ThetaHealing. After taking their first class, they may think that suddenly they are the experts, when really they are just beginning to learn.

Being *confident* is witnessing the Creator of All That Is doing the healings and being *egotistical* is taking the credit for the healings. It is important to know the difference between these two very separate concepts.

FREE YOUR MIND

I believe if we can maintain and focus the right combinations of virtues, in the right formulas, even for a few seconds, we can move and fold the universe and transport ourselves from one planet to another. However, many people, upon being presented with this possibility, take on a heavy emotion in order keep themselves grounded in this reality and stay where they are. We create these feelings so that we don't have to take the next step in our spiritual evolution. This is why it is important to be aware of when we are tapping into negative feelings and consciously refocus our thoughts. (This doesn't mean that we should be angry with ourselves for having these feelings, only that we should refocus.)

Anytime that we become obsessed with negative feelings about a situation or a person, these feelings are keeping us in a 'safe zone.' What does this mean? It may be that our ancestors never went beyond a certain point of development in their DNA. If we go beyond this 'safe zone' in the DNA, we will change not only our own lives, but the lives of those ancestors as well. Everything that we accomplish in this life is projected in some way backward and forward in our genetic DNA through the morphogenetic field. By changing our DNA, we can change thousands of people in the future and the past. This means that the things that we do in this lifetime matter in ways of which we may be completely unaware. It also means that the emotional component of our DNA can be our enemy or our friend, depending on our awareness of it.

While it is important to clear negative beliefs in the DNA, it is also important to develop the virtues that are needed to work with a Law, for instance in bending time or moving matter, as these trigger healing or further progress.

Even Fifth-Plane masters still have to progress on all the planes of existence. So, lessons are brought into our life in order to teach us the virtues we need to work with the Laws. We have within us the knowledge of which virtues we must master on this plane. And what we can do here is limitless as long as we keep moving forward.

In order to bend the Laws of the universe, we must first connect with the Seventh Plane Energy of All That Is with the realization that we are connected to everything. The way that we reach this realization is by using the Theta brainwave and experiencing the pure energy of love.

When we realize that we are not separate from the Creator, we can direct our thoughts. We can go through the universe if those thoughts are backed by virtues such as kindness and love. But if our thoughts are backed by resentment, they cannot travel through the universe at faster than light speed.

The first step is to know the All That Is Energy. Once we realize that we are part of this energy, we can focus our thoughts on what we want to have done. We go up and connect to the Creator and focus. It is all about focus. And the only way that we can maintain this focus is by having the virtues and attributes that are needed for it.

This is all intertwined with our divine timing, our mission on this planet. Whatever it is that we want to learn on this planet, we will create instances in which to learn it. For instance, if we want to have strength, we will create situations in which strength is needed.

Our subconscious and the divine timing of our soul are fully aware of our interaction with the planes of existence and our need to develop a particular virtue. They already know what attributes we are seeking. So it is important to explore what is going on in our life, to ascertain what we are creating and to avoid allowing our subconscious to run wild and create adventures in order to acquire certain attributes.

ACQUIRING VIRTUES (IN THE HIGHEST AND BEST WAY)

1. Ask yourself the following questions:

   'What's going in my life?'

   'What challenges am I having?'

   'Why am I having these challenges and are they being created so that I can acquire virtues or do I have to work on my beliefs?'

   'What virtues am I learning? What virtues am I currently working on to attain mastership and gain knowledge of a Law?'

   'Have I mastered the virtues I'm currently working on?'

2. In order to have the full complement of attributes to acquire a virtue, you should go up to the Seventh Plane (*see pages 13 and 14*) and ask the Creator to download into you the attributes you lack.

3. Ask yourself: 'Am I afraid of acquiring new virtues?'

4. Write down what you fear, so that you can release it.

5. How would you like to have every virtue that you already have magnified 10 times? Write down the virtues you already have and the virtues you'd like to magnify.

6. Write down which Laws you have the ability to bend.

7. Is your ego your friend or is it out of control?

Downloads for Virtues (i.e., go to the Seventh Plane and ask for these traits)

'I am able to be kind.'

'Everywhere I go, I shine with God's pearlescent light.'

'I radiate compassion.'

'I radiate kindness.'

'I radiate a high vibration of humor.'

Applying the Positive

In the development of ThetaHealing, one of the most important things we have learned is that we create learning opportunities not only from negative beliefs, but from positive ones as well. *But if we don't grasp the positive and apply it in our life, it is likely that we will keep recycling the negative over and over again.*

Our negative beliefs were created because they served us, and on some level we wanted them to. So it is imperative that we are conscious of our projected thought-forms while in a Theta state. This is why it is important to use belief work to remove and replace negative programs in addition to downloading feelings from the Creator to bring us to a place of purity in our thoughts.

In belief work we find the negative bottom belief and see how it is serving us and what we are getting out of it. It is important to realize what we have learned from it, so that we can go forward and clear it.

BELIEF WORK ON THE IMPOSSIBLE

It may take some belief work to change what you believe to be impossible. But clearing beliefs pertaining to what is perceived as impossible will free your mind from the chains that bind you to the group consciousness of the Third Plane. To some people, it is impossible to heal another person with a thought.

Energy test for:

'It is impossible to heal with the power of thought.'

'It is impossible to connect to the Laws.'

'It is impossible to bend the Laws.'

'It is impossible to attain virtues.'

'It is impossible to free my mind.'

'It is impossible to develop psychic abilities.'

41

DEVELOPING ABILITIES THROUGH VIRTUES

What would you be able to do if you could hold the vibration of multiple virtues for hours or even days at a time? Ask yourself what would happen if you stepped into all of your abilities. Would your vibration be so high that you would step out of this third-dimensional world and return to the place that you came from? You may find that you have a fear of this. This has no foundation to it, though, because you would not go home to the Fifth Plane unless you had finished what you came here to do.

Here on the Third Plane there are many abilities to develop. We can retrieve abilities from our DNA, from a past life, or from a different time or place. Healing and shamanic abilities are handed down through the DNA; however, empathic healing and emotional healing are abilities that still have to be refined. Some abilities are sent down through genetics, but we also bring with us abilities that are carried by the soul-energy. I know that I brought ancient knowledge with me when I came here that is spiritual in nature. I came into this life with the knowledge how to connect to my heavenly father and heavenly mother. I know that I've taught ThetaHealing before. When I'm teaching it now there are times when the information comes out spontaneously because I already know it.

It may be that our ancestors were great healers who were tortured or killed for their talents. We may be able to heal, but these ancestral fears may be stopping us from reaching our full potential. Eliminating this fear may help reveal these healing abilities. I always tune my energy to the tingly white light of the Seventh Plane so that I don't carry any fear. When you visualize yourself as that tingly white light, fear is gone.

There are many abilities and attributes that some people consider to be negative in nature, but we should be careful about this. For instance, being stubborn is not a bad ability and neither is being confident.

With any ability that we bring forward into this life, it is important to bring the wisdom of how to use it as well. Think about the abilities you have brought with you on a spiritual level. For instance, with clairvoyance, you may be able to read someone's thoughts, but being able to read someone's heart is completely different. When you can read someone's heart, it gives you the ability to see into their life.

Other abilities are slowing down time, being able to witness a healing and one of the most important of all, kindness.

Kindness

I was born with kindness and I see the same attribute in some of my grandchildren. You can see in their eyes that compassion is in the depths of their soul. Every once in a while you can see them give you a look of compassion and pity when they see the deviations of the human condition.

I once had an interesting telepathic conversation with my nine-month-old grandson. We started to jabber back and forth in baby talk and then we started to laugh. He was explaining to me how funny humans looked to him. He told me how hilarious we were when we thought so highly of ourselves and drove our cars and took ourselves so seriously. He observed how dramatic we could be as adults and how we wasted so much time on silly endeavors. He told me how cool it was to be able to move his body. He projected this energy with love and kindness instead of ridicule. He had the wisdom of 1,000 years inside his tiny little body. Where did this wisdom and kindness come from? From his soul and his DNA.

This type of empathic kindness was always easy for me too. If you are like this, though, you don't always say what is on your mind and you sit in the corner because you don't want say anything that will hurt someone's feelings. This is because you can literally feel another person's feelings. This ability is important when you are a healer.

Healing

There is a reason why some people are better healers than others and this is because they possess the virtues they need to make the healings happen.

When someone asks to be a better healer, all their fears, doubts and disbeliefs come up to be cleared, because these are the negative beliefs that will stop them. If they don't realize that this is what is going on, the clearing process can be a challenge.

A woman came to me in one of my classes and said, 'Vianna, I asked God to be a better healer and now I don't want anything to do with healing

43

anymore. When I got home, all my family members got sick and I had to work on all of them!'

She had asked to become a better healer and the best way to do that is to work with people. So God gave her lots of people to practice on.

These are the kind of little lessons that might come into your life. The soul already knows what it wants and what it needs to grow. So the people who come into your life might be there to teach you the virtues of patience, compassion, and forgiveness, even though they are making you miserable. But if these attributes are mastered, then you can move to a better vibration in life. Instead of becoming miserable, you can realize that these situations are opportunities to learn. Then you can release yourself from the need to be taught through drama.

In a healing, you cannot be judgmental or critical toward the person being healed and you have to be able to treat them with compassion. So if you refine these attributes, your healing abilities will blossom.

When I started to teach, I soon came to the realization that everyone comes to learn ThetaHealing for different reasons. Some people learn the modality and don't do healings professionally. Some people come to heal their body. They heal their body, they heal a few friends and relatives, and that is the extent of their use of ThetaHealing. Some people learn how to teach the modality to others and don't do healings on a regular basis.

Looking at my students in this light, there is a reason why some people can use the methods that I teach and why some people cannot. Much of this is because they don't work with enough people to get the proficiency that they need. I have worked with thousands of people in thousands of different situations over the years, and not everyone has the opportunity to have this kind of experience. But working in service with people is only part of the answer. The other side of the sacred coin is communicating with the divine, and this is where the seven planes of existence come in.

In my first books I teach that you can go up and connect with the divine. ThetaHealing is about communicating with the divine in the service of others. Communicating with the divine and reaching the divine should be the first goal of a good ThetaHealer. But for the student who wants to continue to develop their healing abilities, ThetaHealing has so much more to offer.

One of the conversations that I had with God was about witnessing a healing. I asked, 'Why can't everyone witness a healing? After all, it is their birthright.'

God told me, 'Vianna it is because they lack kindness. Kindness is a key to being able to heal.'

Then I explored the question why are some people good healers and other people not so good at it? I found that some people had a decent grasp of healing work but for some reason they just couldn't apply it. They blamed God, they blamed their clients, and then they blamed their teacher. They failed to recognize that the cause was their own thoughts, or the thoughts that they were missing.

Another mistake, as we have seen, is when a student thinks that they are the Creator and they are doing the healings and readings. When they think like this, they will ultimately be unsuccessful when they really need to succeed.

In order to witness and therefore accomplish a healing, you have to master *restraint*. Can you think back to all the times when you wanted to punch someone in the nose but you didn't? On your healing journey there will be times when you will feel like giving people a piece of your mind, and this will change your vibration. In order to be able to heal you have to have compassion. Compassion is a Law, but it is also a virtue.

Faith in the Healing

We had just moved into our house in Kalispell, Montana, and my daughter Bobbi had brought my grandchildren over to share in the excitement of the new place. There were still boxes everywhere and the house was in disarray. The little boys were full of energy and began exuberantly to explore every nook and cranny of the house. They focused on a storage room upstairs, which made a perfect place to for them to play. They had been frolicking happily for some time when suddenly my oldest grandson, Remington, came charging downstairs, his eyes swollen almost shut and covered with hives.

I was terrified because I knew he could go into anaphylactic shock. I told Bobbi, 'Hurry! Get him in the car and let's go to the hospital!'

But she calmly looked at me and said, 'Don't worry, Momma, it will be all right. We don't have time for that. Just do a healing on him.'

So I calmed down and went up to witness a healing on little Remington. After several minutes, the swelling began to dissipate. As time went on, it went down completely and Remington was fine. Apparently it was something in the carpet in the storage room that had caused the allergic reaction. I'd never seen a reaction come on or disappear as quickly as this one had, but what was truly amazing was the pure faith of Bobbi in her mother.

For a healing to happen, you need a little bit of faith. This is why ThetaHealing works with other modalities and religions – it lets you keep your faith. You take that faith and use it. Having faith in a loving God is allowing something to happen instead of blocking it. You also have to possess the virtue of gratitude – being thankful. You have to have wonder, and God's definition of hope and service. You have to be in service to your fellow man (or woman) in order for a healing to work. If the healings are not happening, then it is from the lack of one of these attributes.

Of course we can't make someone heal if they don't want to heal, even from their own physical or mental destruction. With some people, there is something inside them that does not want to accept a healing. Accepting this can be difficult for some healers. But if we download the client with faith, kindness, and forgiveness before we do a healing, our chances of an instantaneous healing will be much better.

The kind of mood that we are in as a healer is also very important. If we go up and ask for an extra dose of faith, kindness, and forgiveness before we do a healing, this will also change the outcome. All of these things need to be present each and every time, and this may be why healings don't always work.

On the other side of the sacred coin, the healings might be working great and then all of a sudden you get in a fight with your wife, your husband, your mother, or your boss. Then the healings just don't happen. This means that other aspects have sneaked into your life and changed your vibration. Things have sneaked into your healing that I talked about in my first book, and these are resentment, fear, doubt, and disbelief.

In order to do a healing you must be cleared of resentment. This doesn't mean that you have to be *completely* cleared of resentment, just that at the moment of healing there cannot be any anger or resentment in your space.

You have to be able to go up and connect in a peaceful moment of pure love. We are entitled to use this energy of love, but we have to be able to maintain the essence of it.

With practice, you can make this virtuous connection stronger and stronger. The more these positive feelings interplay in your life, the less the negative feelings can pull you down.

You must first connect to the energy of All That Is. When you realize that you're not separate, the Creator will show you how to witness a healing. Then you can go up and witness a healing, but you must have the virtues to direct your thoughts to accomplish the healing. It is everyone's birthright to witness a healing and you only have to hold the energy of purity for a split second. But in order to do this you have to hold the All That Is energy and the energy of the correct virtue for that split second. So you have to know the virtue and incorporate it into your life in order to use it in a healing. And when you acquire a virtue, you have to keep it activated for the rest of your life.

Even though it is God who does the healing, as the healer I am the witness that makes it possible through the act of co-creation. One of the reasons that I can witness healings is because I have faith that it can be done, but, as we know, I also have something that is very important: kindness. I was born with kindness. I know how to be kind. If you are not kind, then you are not going to be a good healer. So, if you want to be a better healer and pray to be better at it, God will set up a training program to show you how to be kind, or to learn compassion, or to acquire whatever attribute you need to access the Law of Healing.

In order to facilitate a healing in another person you only have to create a small space in their brain by pulling out enough resentment for it to work. This creates a small opening in the time–space continuum.

With the knowledge that you must have certain virtues to be a better healer, the next step is to stop and look at the stresses in your life that might be blocking a healing.

The Law of Healing is the vibration of free will. The Law of Free Will is a Law of the universe that cannot be broken. *It just is.* So another thing to know about healing is that people have free will. This means that we cannot do anything for a person without their permission. If you are reading this book with other ideas in mind, perhaps this information is not for you. Anyone who abuses this work must understand that there are other Laws that are connected to Free Will, such as the Law of Truth and the Law of Justice. To break the imperative of a Law such as Free Will would mean to be in direct opposition to these Laws. And they work synergistically with one another to enhance the attributes that are inherent in each.

In fact the best way to lose your gift of healing is to start doing two things in spiritual healing work. One is to deny that there is a God or All That Is energy. The other is to interfere with another person's free agency and force your will upon the world or upon others. Forcing your spiritual patterns upon others will only make you *think* you are becoming powerful. What will happen is that any gift that you might have will be lessened or distorted.

All Laws must be activated through the Seventh Plane as well as with the appropriate virtues. The virtues needed for healing are: acceptance, compassion, courage, faith, forgiveness, gratitude, hope, kindness, restraint, service, and wonder.

This means that you have true compassion for what is happening to the client without being overwhelmed by the poignancy of their situation. It also means that you must be able to maintain these virtues as thought-forms for long enough for the healing to happen.

Psychic Ability

The ability to connect to the Creator is our birthright and some people are born psychics, but they still have to develop and practice their talents. Some people stop their psychic abilities when they are young and it is only when they are older that they begin to develop them again. All abilities have to be practiced.

Generally, psychic ability skips generations unless both parents are strongly psychic and have recessive genes that carry the predisposition. Many people may have these psychic sides lying dormant in their DNA.

In a psychic reading you have to train yourself to be right. Don't let anyone program you that it is all right to be wrong. Never program anyone that they don't have to be right all the time. Program them that it is right to be correct all the time. I have heard a lot of psychics say that they are right 10 percent of the time, but a psychic should be right most of the time. A good psychic should be clear at least 91.3 percent of the time, and 97 percent if they have practiced for more than three years.

Why do some people have psychic abilities and others don't? It is because their thought-patterns are different than those of other people. Do you accept what other people define as reality or do you go your own way? A good psychic goes their own way.

When I first did psychic readings, I locked myself in a room and did 18 to 20 readings a day so that I could learn what I am telling you in this book. It would have been easier had I known the right questions to ask the Creator. Even then, though, you may not understand some of the answers and messages that you get, at least at first.

When I first became aware of this path that I am now on, I began to get premonitions of the future. In one of these premonitions I saw myself underneath a pyramid in a cave. I thought that this was unlikely, but many years later, when I first went to Mexico, I had the opportunity to go into the caves underneath the Temple of the Sun at Teotihuacan that the general public is not allowed to see. When this happened to me, the premonition finally made sense.

This premonition was about the future in this life. What is important with premonitions is knowing where they are coming from. The question you should ask is, 'Is this coming from the past, from the DNA, or from the future?' A good psychic is able to distinguish between all their past, present and future lives within the context of this lifetime.

Being a good psychic means seeing the truth, having kindness, exercising understanding, and having tolerance. Tolerance is a major virtue here, because you may not like what you find in someone's mind.

THE SECRET RECIPE FOR ACQUIRING ABILITIES AND WORKING WITH LAWS

What virtues do you need to master in order to acquire particular abilities? The following is a list of abilities and the virtues required.

The Ability to Be Ageless

It's amazing that we can focus our thoughts and heal the body of sickness, but most of us stop there. The next step should be to focus our thoughts on telling the body to be persistently well, strong, and ageless. These things can bring about a healthy body. To be truly healthy takes another set of virtues.

Virtues required: The Law of Time governs the ability to be ageless, so all the virtues of the Law of Time are required: kindness, love, pure intent, reverence, sincerity, trust, vision, and wonder.

Blocks: Fear and hopelessness.

The Ability to Be Psychic

Virtues required: Kindness, tolerance, truthfulness, and understanding. (Remember that tolerance is a major virtue here, because you may not like what you find in someone's mind.)

Blocks: Resentment.

The Ability to Heal

Virtues required: Acceptance, courage, compassion, faith, forgiveness, gratitude, hope, kindness, restraint, service, and wonder.

Blocks: Disbelief, doubt, and fear,

The Ability to Manifest Instantly

Manifesting things instantly means that you have an understanding of the Law of Illusion.

Virtues required: The virtues for the Law of Attraction, the Law of Illusion, and the Law of Vibration: acceptance, creativity, detachment, determination, fairness, faith, focus, forgiveness, hope, humor, imagination, joy, love, loyalty, mercy, nobility, pure intent, purity of heart, tolerance, trust, wisdom, and wonder.

Blocks: Anger, arrogance, doubt, fear, hate, resentment, and lack of understanding.

The Ability to Master the Elements

The ability to master the elements of earth, air, fire and water are under the Law of Life.

Virtues required: Acceptance, beauty, conviction, curiosity, dedication, focus, honor, love of others, perseverance, pure intent, sincerity, thankfulness, tolerance, and wonder.

Blocks: Egotism.

The Ability to Produce Art and Music

The Law of Light and the Law of Vibration govern artistic and musical ability. Art and Music are Sub-Laws.

Virtues required: Creativity, enthusiasm, focus, imagination, patience, and vision.

Blocks: Fear.

The Ability to Read Minds

I believe that in ancient times we were able to talk to one another with the power of pure thought. When we come into this world as a tiny baby, we're still able to understand others in this way. But in order to survive the negativity that we're bombarded with, we stop doing it. As we grow older, our brain still has the ability to do it, but we don't use it anymore.

Virtues required: The ability to read minds is governed by the Law of Truth, so all the virtues of this Law are required: commitment, compassion, faith, patience, tolerance, and understanding.

Blocks: Egotism, remorse, resentment, and the desire for revenge.

The Ability to See the Future

The ability to see the future is governed by the Law of Attraction, the Law of Time, and the Hall of Records.

Virtues required: Compassion, dedication, devotion, kindness, loyalty, service, tolerance, trust, vision, and wisdom.

Blocks: Fear.

The Ability to See Truth in Another Person

The ability to see truth in another person involves being able to see and read into their heart. All I have to do is to look at what is going on in someone's heart and I can see what they are up to and hear what they are thinking.

Virtues required: Compassion, kindness, tolerance, truthfulness, and understanding.

Blocks: Jealousy and resentment.

The Ability to Teleport

Virtues required: The virtues required for teleportation are the virtues for the Laws of Time and Vibration: acceptance, creativity, detachment, determination, fairness, faith, focus, forgiveness, hope, humor, imagination, joy, kindness, love, loyalty, mercy, nobility, pure intent, purity of heart, reverence, sincerity, tolerance, trust, vision, wisdom, and wonder.

Blocks: Criticism, egotism, and fear.

THE LAWS AND THEIR VIRTUES

The Law of Action

Virtues required: Courage, hope, love, and patience.

Blocks: Complaining, fear, laziness, and whining.

The Law of Attraction

Virtues required: Acceptance, creativity, detachment, determination, fairness, faith, focus, forgiveness, hope, humor, imagination, joy, kindness, love, loyalty, mercy, nobility, pure intent, purity of heart, tolerance, trust, wisdom, and wonder.

Blocks: Anger, arrogance, doubt, fear, hate, resentment, and lack of understanding.

The Law of Balance

Virtues required: Acceptance, courage, flexibility, forgiveness, gratitude, love, passion, patience, reverence, tolerance, understanding, and wisdom.

Blocks: Criticism and egotism.

The Law of Cause and Effect (Law of Karma)

My girlfriend decided to call in the Law of Karma on her son, who was up to mischief. When she did this, he was arrested. This is because the Law of Karma had activated the Law of Justice. So he had to pay a fine – or, rather, she had to pay it for him, since he was underage. He was then released into her custody, so the justice system ended up having a great deal of control over her life. Karma is connected to the Law of Justice and the Law of DNA, so what affected her son was going to affect her. This is why you should be careful when you call in this Law. You should be spotlessly clean when you do so. It may affect you in ways you're not prepared for.

Belief work can process the virtues for this Law very quickly.

Virtues required: Belief, compassion, detachment, determination, devotion, forgiveness, humility, imagination, joy, kindness, love, pure intent, service, truthfulness, wisdom, and wonder.

Blocks: Attachment to false beliefs and false suffering, conceit, fear of moving forward, forcefulness, and pride (in the negative sense).

The Law of Compassion

The Law of Compassion is a powerful etheric Law that, once mastered, can bend many of the other Laws.

Virtues required: Love, patience, service, tolerance, and understanding.

Blocks: Blind arrogance.

The Law of Dimensions

The Law of Dimensions is under the Law of Time. Using it can move you from one place to another through tiny black holes.

Virtues required: Bravery, confidence, courage, dignity, faith, forgiveness, imagination, kindness, love, loyalty, and vision.

Blocks: Anger, hate, and the desire for revenge.

The Law of DNA

Virtues required: Acceptance, authenticity, commitment, cooperation, courage, honor, love, respect, and understanding.

Blocks: Regret and resentment.

The Law of Electricity

Virtues required: Cleverness, confidence, dedication, determination, intelligence, love, loyalty, modesty, and self-discipline.

Blocks: Resentment.

The Law of the Elements

This Law encompasses each element of the periodic table. It is under the Law of Nature. It is possible to change the atomic structure of matter with this Law.

Virtues required: Action, belief, faith, focus, and pure intent.

Blocks: Disruption, lack of respect, and selfishness.

The Law of Emotion

Virtues required: Compassion, humility, love, pure intent, and purpose.

Blocks: Depression, fear, hatred, resentment, and sadness.

The Law of Focus

Virtues required: Love, perseverance, and pure intent.

Blocks: Fear and resentment.

The Law of Free Agency (or Free Will)

This Law cannot be bent, broken, or influenced.

The Law of Illusion

Virtues required: Acceptance, creativity, detachment, determination, fairness, faith, focus, forgiveness, hope, humor, imagination, joy, kindness, love, loyalty, mercy, nobility, pure intent, purity of heart, tolerance, trust, wisdom, and wonder.

Blocks: Anger, arrogance, doubt, fear, hate, resentment, and lack of understanding.

The Law of Justice

When I called in the Law of Justice to take care of a situation, I didn't realize that it was going to be so slow. If you think that the legal system is slow, you should see the Law of Justice! The Law of Justice works so closely with the Law of Karma that it may be another lifetime before any justice is done. When you call in the Law of Justice it brings justice to all parties concerned, not just one party. Justice is slow in prevailing and by the time it finishes, you may be over the need for it.

Virtues required: Action, forgiveness, hope, imagination, joy, kindness, love, mercy, and pure intent.

Blocks: Resentment and the desire for revenge.

The Law of Life

Virtues required: Acceptance, beauty, conviction, curiosity, dedication, focus, honor, love, perseverance, pure intent, sincerity, thankfulness, tolerance, and wonder.

Blocks: Depression.

The Law of Light

Virtues required: Acceptance, beauty, belief, creativity, hope, joy, love, truthfulness, vision, witnessing, and wonder.

Blocks: Depression, discouragement, fear, sorrow and spitefulness.

The Law of Magnetism

Magnetism is one of the greatest sources of energy. In order to bend this Law you must acquire all the virtues that are listed.

Virtues required: Acceptance, assertiveness, authenticity, beauty, belief, bravery, caring, charisma, clarity, cleanliness, cleverness, commitment, communication, compassion, confidence, consideration, contentment, conviction, cooperation, courage, creativity, curiosity, dedication, detachment, determination, devotion, dignity, discipline, endurance, enthusiasm, excellence, fairness, faith, flexibility, focus, forgiveness, fortitude, friendliness, generosity, gentleness, grace, graciousness, gratitude, harmony, helpfulness, honesty, honor, hope, humility, humor, idealism, imagination, integrity, intelligence, joy, justice, kindness, love, loyalty, mercy, moderation, modesty, morality, nobility, optimism, orderliness, passion, patience, peace, perseverance, playfulness, preparedness, pure intent, purposefulness, reliability, respect, responsibility, reverence, self-discipline, service, sincerity, sympathy, tact, temperance, tenaciousness, thankfulness, tolerance, trust, truthfulness, understanding, unity, vision, wisdom, and wonder.

Blocks: Fear, gossip, and selfishness.

The Law of Motion

Virtues required: Authenticity, bravery, cleverness, courage, curiosity, flexibility, friendliness, love, service, and vision.

Blocks: Forcefulness and jealousy.

The Law of Nature

In order to bend this Law you must acquire all the virtues that are listed. Once you are able to understand the Law of Nature, you will be able to control the weather and the elements of earth, water, fire, and air.

Virtues required: Kindness, love, modesty, nobility, peacefulness, perseverance, pure intent, and sincerity.

Blocks: Discouragement, lack of incentive, and weakness.

The Law of Protection

Virtues required: Forgiveness. (Forgiveness is the highest protection.)

Blocks: Hatred.

The Law of Pure Intent

Virtues required: Clarity, commitment, compassion, forgiveness, graciousness, gratitude, integrity, kindness, love, morality, and patience.

Blocks: Chaos, criticism, and gossip.

The Law of Sacred Geometry

This Law can be used to change atomic structures.

Virtues required: Cleverness, faith, focus, forgiveness, kindness, love, pure intent, respect, trust, understanding, wisdom, and wonder.

Blocks: Fear and selfishness.

The Law of Thought

This is a key Law to open dimensions with the Law of Time. The Law of Thought is not confined to this universe but has a multi-dimensional energy to it.

Virtues required: All the virtues are needed to master this Law.

Blocks: Criticism and fear.

The Law of Time

The Law of Time allows you to stretch or bend time.

Virtues required: Kindness, love, pure intent, reverence, sincerity, trust, vision, and wonder.

Blocks: Doubt and fear.

The Law of Tones

Virtues required: Beauty, belief, creativity, focus, love, reliability, reverence, service, vision, and wonder.

Blocks: Depression, fear, and self-disdain.

The Law of Truth

The Law of Truth is above all the Laws except for the Law of Compassion. If you connect to the Law of Truth and expect it to answer you kindly, you will be sadly disappointed. The answer will be immediate and to the point. You will only get kindness when you go to the Creator and your answer is filtered through the Seventh Plane.

The ability to read people's thoughts is governed by the Law of Truth.

The Law of Truth is an emotional Law. To work with it, you must be born as or be willing to become a seeker of truth.

Virtues required: Commitment, compassion, faith, patience, tolerance, and understanding.

Blocks: Fear, remorse, resentment, and the desire for revenge.

The Law of Velocity

Virtues required: Action, hope, imagination, joy, kindness, love, and pure intent.

Blocks: Criticism and laziness.

The Law of Vibration

Virtues required: Acceptance, creativity, detachment, determination, fairness, faith, focus, forgiveness, hope, humor, imagination, joy, kindness, love, loyalty, mercy, nobility, pure intent, purity of heart, tolerance, trust, wisdom, and wonder.

Blocks: Discouragement.

The Law of Wisdom

Virtues required: Empathy, kindness, love, and understanding.

Blocks: Regret and sorrow.

The Law of Witness

Virtues required: Acceptance, hope, mercy, self-discipline, truthfulness, and trust.

Blocks: Criticism, doubt, and jealousy.

SACRED LANGUAGES
The Sixth Plane of Existence: The Divine Music of All That Is

Everything in creation, from the tiniest particle to the massive expanse of the universe itself, has a sacred language that is a divine music all its own. Every inhabitant of every plane of existence has sacred languages that are musical tones. While this divine music is similar in its context, each aspect of creation emits a slightly different version of it.

There was a time when these languages were common knowledge and the very Earth would speak to us. In this reality of the Third Plane of Existence, there are some people who are connected to the planes of existence in such a way that they still understand these languages. The languages have a thought-form vibration and are inter-dimensional in their composition. There are some words in all of them that are attached to thoughts that have a special effect on the universe. ('Speaking in tongues' is a sacred language and sounds similar to Hebrew or Sanskrit but is not the same as these sacred languages that we are discussing.)

The languages of the Fifth and Sixth Planes of Existence are divine tones and divine music. If you go up to the Sixth Plane of Existence and you hear music, you can ask for clarity so that you can understand the divine language of tones and music.

The universal language is music, tones, and numbers. When you are able to recognize the music in everything and that everything has a tone, you will find it possible to heal with tones.

If you were a being of the Fifth or the Sixth Plane of Existence listening to us talking on the Third Plane of Existence, you would know that we were using a tone of music that was unique to us. Have you noticed that some of our human languages sound much more musical than others? For instance, if you listen to Italian, Spanish or French, they sound very musical. Every one of our languages has a unique vibration. I believe that as these languages developed in different cultures, the brain of the people in those cultures developed differently as well. It has been my observation that people in different cultures process language in different parts of the brain. The brain receives the tones of the language differently. For instance, I believe that Japanese is received at the back of the brain and English is received at the front of the brain.

Just as the DNA in the body emits a divine tone of communication, so the organs of the physical body sing to one another in a sacred language of communication. This divine music is not just within the body, since the body is merely a tiny representation of the cosmos. The cosmos itself uses a similar divine music to communicate. Every world has its own song that it sings to other planets. Every solar system uses its own tones of divine music. Every galaxy has its own special song of communication, and so on and so forth up to the very universe itself, which has its own divine music of tonal communication. Even the essence of light has a tone and a vibration of its own. Each of the planes of existence has its own special music of communication, which it plays to other planes to create a marriage of energy between them.

The Sixth Plane of Existence holds the knowledge of the tones that create balance in the body. It also holds the knowledge of the tones that can change the vibration of any bacterium or virus. It is through the Law of Vibration that we learn the tones and divine music to communicate with the universe.

We may have the program 'that we can only understand the language we are taught as children' so we need to download the knowledge of the true language of divine music of All That Is. This divine musical language is an equation of the Sixth and Seventh Planes of Existence.

SEVENTH-PLANE PROCESS: SACRED LANGUAGES

Virtues required: Fairness, faith, focus, imagination, joy, purity of heart, trust, and wonder.

1. Go up to the Seventh Plane (*see pages 13 and 14*) and make the command, *'Creator of All That Is, it is commanded [or requested] that I understand the sacred languages of the planes of existence. Show me in the highest and best way.'*

2. Witness knowledge of the sacred languages being brought into yourself on all levels of your being.

3. When you have finished, rinse yourself off with Seventh-Plane energy and stay connected to it.

Download for Sacred Languages

'Creator of All That Is, it is commanded [or requested] that
I be downloaded with the understanding of the universal
language of music, tones, and numbers from the Sixth Plane.'

We cannot access the power of the first six planes unless we have a tone or a name, or first go to the Creator. The Creator has access to everything.

If you clean up enough programs from your being and afterward realize that you can bend a spoon, you will then understand the structure of material matter in this Third Plane and how to use more than one plane at a time.

In previous incarnations many of us have been alchemists, shamans, and holy men and women. There are age-old rules and regulations that come with these positions that are connected to the planes of existence. However, if you first go to the Seventh Plane, you can access these energies without abiding by the rules and regulations of the lower planes. You must also understand that something is not made of nothing. Each plane follows this simple rule of Law. On the Seventh Plane of Existence, that 'something' is the All That Is Energy.

Sacred Names

At one time in the distant past we all knew the sacred languages of the planes – the forgotten languages of the minerals, the animals, and the plants. The first step in the rediscovery of these forgotten languages is knowing our sacred name.

Every being of the planes of existence has a sacred name for every plane of existence. Each one of us actually has four possible soul names for each plane. Ask the Creator for your name on each plane of existence and wait for them. If they don't come immediately, wait and trust that they will come. Sometimes people are stressed when they ask for their sacred names and they don't come. Then they come later on that night when they are getting ready for bed.

Remember that some of these names will be perceived as tones or will be heard in a musical form that changes a person's frequency of vibration.

Once you find your sacred names, I don't suggest that you share them with everyone around you. Giving everyone the knowledge of your sacred names is not a good idea, because they are sacred to you. It is not a good idea to put them on your calling card and give them out.

Your sacred name is a large part of your natural vibration. If you have an understanding of someone's vibration you can do amazing things. You can send what I call the fallen to the light with the use of their sacred name. You find out what this is by asking the Creator for it.

It works the same way with bacteria and viruses. Everything in nature has its own vibration and if you know what that vibration is, you can use it. When you understand the vibration signature of a virus by way of its sacred name, for example, you can change the virus.

There was a time when I thought that the best way to deal with viruses was to find a way to destroy them. I would ask the Creator for the opposite vibration to a particular virus and use it to make the virus disappear. This only worked part of the time. Then the Creator showed me a better way: changing the beliefs we have that are drawing the virus to us and then changing them in the virus. This is so the virus can evolve into a higher intelligence and be less harmful. I learned that, like all life, viruses and bacteria serve a purpose, and this purpose can be elevated with belief work. There may come a day when doctors use viruses as a delivery system for some kinds of medicine.

To change the vibration of disease into something that is harmless through a tone from the Sixth Plane, use the following exercise:

SEND A TONE FROM THE SIXTH PLANE OF EXISTENCE

In this exercise you go up to the Seventh Plane and then connect to the Sixth Plane to send a tone through a person to stop bad bacteria or a bad virus and heal the person.

It is better, however, to change a person's beliefs so that they don't attract a virus in the first place. As their beliefs change, the vibration of their own tone will change as well. So use this exercise only in an emergency.

Virtues required: Acceptance, compassion, courage, fairness, faith, forgiveness, gratitude, hope, imagination, joy, kindness, purity of heart, restraint, service, trust, and wonder.

1. Go up to the Seventh Plane (*see pages 13 and 14*) and make the command: *'Creator of All That Is, it is commanded [or requested] to connect with the Sixth Plane of Existence and the Law of Magnetism to send a tone for [name purpose]. Thank you. It is done, it is done, it is done.'*

2. Witness the tone being sent for that purpose and continue watching until the process is finished.

3. Rinse yourself off with Seventh-Plane energy and stay connected to it.

All Laws have their own sacred name that designates their vibration. Once you have mastered the abilities and virtues that are needed to access a Law, it is necessary to know the sacred name of that Law. This sacred name is the pure quintessence of the Law that is the vibration-intonation to awaken and direct it for the intended purpose. Once the virtues to master a Law have been acquired, asking to know the sacred name of the Law is the last step to truly knowing how to activate it.

DOWNLOADING VIBRATIONS FROM THE LAWS

The essence of life is vibration. What is important is to be able to recognize and download knowledge of these vibrations for the enrichment of our lives. For instance, if I were an artist, I would want to download from the Creator knowledge of the vibration to give people divine inspiration through my paintings. If I were a musician, I would want to download my instrument and myself with the vibration of being able to inspire joy in the people who listened to me. If I were an inventor, I would want to know everything there was to know about the vibration of the Laws that would enable me to create incredible things. You have the knowledge of the universal vibration at your fingertips through the Seventh Plane of Existence and the Laws.

The Vibration of Color

Everything living thing that has color has an essence, an energy, associated with it. For instance, being surrounded by trees gives us a feeling of wellbeing that cannot be explained. Most trees are green and the vibration of this color gives out a healing energy that surrounds us as it creates the oxygen that gives us life. The color green is the vibration of many plants and trees that have healing components to them by way of herbal medicines.

Just like plants and trees, we have a color scheme within us as well. One of our missions in this life is to focus our energy on creating attributes and virtues to make our color pure. As we acquire each virtue, we acquire a different array of the colors of the rainbow spectrum. Once we have all these colors working in equal amounts, they converge into that tingly white energy of perfection of thought. This is the energy of creation, that essence of pure love of the Seventh Plane.

When we are born, we come onto this plane carrying a pure state of love from an extra-dimensional energy with a color that is pure white with a touch of pink in it. This is because as a baby we have a perfect balance of color, emotion, and love. It is this same tingly white energy that we want to reach in order to be connected to the Creator of All That Is. It is a conversion of every other color into perfect balance. The only other times when we have a white aura are when we are close to death or when we are in intense pain.

As we grow older and experience the negative thoughts of this plane, our aura starts to change to different colors. We only have three main sequences of light; red, green and blue, which mix to create all the other variations. However, if all these aura colors were mixed together, the color that they become would be white.

Our goal is to change enough of our beliefs so that our aura is a tingly white energy. Ultimately, the perfect color is white, which is the iridescent light of All That Is. It is this light that can harmonize the whole body.

The reason that color is important is because it helps us to acquire virtues. This is because each color has attributes that it brings to the table and each color helps to balance the body and mind in a different way. When the body is balanced, it is healthy in spirit, mind, and body.

In the same way, all the virtues converge upon each other to create the same kind of perfection. This is why we have had to focus on adding virtues each lifetime. Many of us have added only three or four virtues each lifetime, but now we have the opportunity to add them all in this space and time.

SEE THE AURA

1. To see someone's aura, start by taking a piece of white paper and putting a dot on the paper.

2. Put your hand down with the dot between your fingers.

3. Concentrate on that dot.

4. As you focus on it, you will see white energy flowing round your fingers. This is your aura.

Once you get used to this and can see the white aura around a person, if you concentrate on it and then look just outside it, you will be able to see the color of their aura. It is pencil-thin around the white. This aura color will change with their mood.

When you take a picture with a Kirlian aura machine, the average person has the same aura color every time. This changes when you connect to the Creator. As you become more spiritually aware and become a rainbow child, your aura color can change from picture to picture. Over time, you begin to get control of the color that you are sending out to the world. You aura also begins to expand as you grow spiritually.

Each of us has our own sequence of colors and these are represented in the aura we bring to the world. But when we access and use the Law of Color and Vibration, the color of our chakras can change along with the color of our aura.

Rainbow children have all the colors in their aura and this means that they have the ability to mix them together to make tingly white. Rainbow children are special children who have come into this existence to change the world. The world has been instinctively waiting for special children to take it into a new age. Some have called them violet-colored or indigos, others have talked about crystal children. To me, the world has been waiting for rainbow children – and they are here now. Whatever we call these enlightened people, they can move energy to create change in the world. A crystal person reflects the energy of anyone in a room, but a rainbow person can *change* the energy of anyone in a room. A rainbow person can do healings. A perfect rainbow person can reach out and change the soul of anyone. We are all evolving into rainbow people.

LIFE LESSONS

Because there are no mistakes in the universe, the experience that you are having has a purpose. Everything in your life is like a fire that is used to forge the soul the way that it should be. You will come to the realization that you are not angry with God or the universe for these life lessons.

The more that you are within the Seventh-Plane energy of pure love, the more virtues you will master just from the vibration of being in it. The ultimate goal is to live your life connected to the Seventh Plane.

But when you come back into the comfort zone of this reality, you may permit yourself to have heavy thoughts once again. This is because your subconscious mind is hardwired to keep you on this plane. This is also why after you have been in the bliss of the Seventh Plane and you come back into Third-Plane reality, you create an argument with your wife or husband, you get angry with your children, or you become angry with yourself – anything to keep yourself in this Third-Plane reality.

LIFE LESSON BELIEF WORK

Sit down with a partner and tell them what is going on in your life.

Follow the thread of belief work to see how any difficult situation in your life is serving you and what it is teaching you.

Your partner may ask:

- 'What is going on in your life and what it is doing to help you grow?'

- 'What are you getting out of the situation and what are you learning from it? What good are you getting out of it?'

- 'What is the biggest challenge in your life?'

- 'Do you feel loved enough?'

- 'Whatever is happing in your life is teaching you something. How are the negative situations (or positive situations) helping you to release vices and acquire virtues?'

VIRTUE BELIEF WORK

Pair up with another person and take turns sharing what is going on in your life and what you have learned from these experiences. With each experience, talk about which virtue you have gained by it.

Explore to find out what virtues you possess already.

BELIEF WORK: 'I HAVE PLENTY'

One of the most important words to use in your life is 'plenty.' Download yourself with the programs 'There is plenty' and 'I have plenty.' Instead of perceiving things in life as being empty, perceive them as being full.

When I didn't have much money, I was worried about my children having enough clothes to wear. However, they always had plenty of clothes because I said, 'We have plenty.' I've used that ever since as one of my mantras.

Energy test for:

'I have plenty.'

'There is plenty.'

'There are plenty of clients.'

'There are plenty of students.'

'There is plenty of money.'

VORTICES AND PORTALS

Vortex Energy

A vortex is spinning electromagnetic activity that can cause a portal to be formed. When combinations of metals are in one place in the Earth, an electromagnetic field can create vortex energy.

Vortex energy can be artificially created with ceremony or by making a sacred site such as a labyrinth or stone circle.

When psychic abilities are balanced, some intuitive people are naturally inclined to create controlled electromagnetic activity that forms vortices and portals of energy. Healers who often go to the Seventh Plane become walking, talking portals. Vortex energy will attract wayward spirits (*see page 120*) and other energies such as UFO experiences. This may be the reason why spirits are drawn to psychics who naturally create vortices.

If a vortex has a negative energy, charging it with a positive energy can change it.

Crystals can cause vortex energy to form. I have put enough crystals in my house to create vortex energy because I like it.

Portals

A portal is different than a vortex. A vortex is swirling electromagnetic energy. A portal is an inter-dimensional tunnel of energy that runs through time and space. Portals are everywhere. If you were to find the right portal, you would be able to go to another planet or dimension.

Spiritual Portals

When a vortex leaves this third dimension and goes all the way through to the fourth or fifth dimension, it creates a spiritual portal. When you go to the Seventh Plane, you are creating your own little spiritual portal. In order for a multi-dimensional spirit to come into a human body, it has to go through a spiritual portal.

Every one of us has a spiritual portal that leads to the Creator of All That Is. When a person dies and their spirit leaves their physical body, it follows this portal to the energy of God's light and from that point it naturally goes to the place on the planes of existence where it belongs. We also use our spiritual portal to send wayward spirits to God's light.

Fairy Portals

The energy emitted by trees and plants can create portals. Fairies use this energy to create portals to other dimensions. (*For more on fairies, see Chapter 7.*)

Bend in Time

A vortex can create a portal that is called a 'bend in time.' This is an imprint of an event in the past that recurs in this time again and again. It happens when certain conditions permit it to manifest. I like vortex energy so much that I once created a bend in time in my house.

When many people die at one time and place, a bend in time can be formed. This is because of the energy that is emitted by the sudden release of the life-force leaving the body. A bend in time cannot be sent to the light like a wayward spirit, but it can be moved.

Sometimes a psychic needs to move a vortex out of the house into the backyard because of the portals that it creates. You cannot shut a vortex, but many psychics try to. They might command the energy to shut down, but once this is done the vortex becomes like a volcano that blows open. This is why it is best to move it a few feet outside the door.

The Portal in Idaho

In 2011, I was told that I would buy a cabin in Island Park, Idaho, the next year just before the month of June. Island Park is in the Targhee National Forest in the mountains above the Snake River Valley and shares the same mountain chain that leads onward to Yellowstone National Park. This place was close to a power spot of mine.

I was spiritually guided to buy the cabin to have a place of tranquility in which I could channel the information for this book. It was also supposed to be a place where I could rest and charge my mind and body with the energy of the mountains. I was told where it would be and, after some searching, I found it. But actually purchasing the place the same year become difficult. It took some months for the person who was selling the place to let it go.

The cabin was exactly where I'd seen it would be, but when I first moved in it was difficult to sleep through the night there without having some kind of bad dream. Going to sleep in this cabin was the strangest thing that had ever happened to me.

After a few nights of this I realized there was a giant vortex of energy right beside my bed. In the middle of the night a portal would open and pull all kinds of weird creatures through it. A definite feeling of evil pervaded the cabin every time that portal was open. I thought to myself, *The Creator should be able to change this portal.*

I knew that vortices were sometimes caused by minerals in the Earth or the past energies of people and I thought that this one could have been created by the people who had owned the cabin before I lived in it. They had experienced so much conflict in their relationship and had deceived each other so many times that a divorce had ensued.

Thinking that this might be the cause, I cleared the cabin of their energy and assumed that this would clear the vortex as well. But in the middle of the night raging energy still came into the cabin by my bed, waking me from a quiet sleep.

On the third night of this weirdness, I was sleeping peacefully when I had a strange dream. A negative entity came to me through the portal and told me that I had to leave my cabin. Of course I told it that it would be the one who left and went up the Creator and commanded that it be gone.

When I did this, the fight was on between us! I found myself being pulled out of my body and my little dog Jasmine started barking at this thing that was attacking me. I woke up and my spirit fell back into my body. This entity wasn't participating in my agenda of sending it to the light! I sent it to the light while I was in a waking state and it went away (or so I thought). But the next morning, it was back in force. Obviously, there was more going on than I'd first thought.

That evening, I had a chat with the Creator about my dilemma. I said, 'Creator, this place is such an inspiration to me in the daytime. I am inspired, I have past-life memories, and I get information about the planes of existence. How can I get rid of this portal?'

The Creator told me, 'Vianna, this portal leads through space and time. It is connected to another galaxy that is filled with negativity. Move it to another place.'

So I went up above my space and commanded that the hole through space be moved outside the cabin to another hill. This worked for a day, but then it was back in the same place again.

I asked God, 'What am I doing wrong?'

God said, 'Vianna, you are misunderstanding me. You need to move the portal's point of origin to a place that has positive energy.'

So I left the portal by the side of my bed and went up through space and time to the point of origin of the portal. I went to the galaxy where negative energy was pouring into the opening of the portal. I witnessed the opening being moved through time and space to another planetary energy that was good for me. Moving the whole thing took an effort of kindness and love, along with total confidence that it could be done. I moved it to a place that was more familiar to me, the Pleiades constellation. I have always been comfortable with the energy coming from there.

After that, the energy of the portal still came into my room, but this time it was good energy that consisted of enlightenment and knowledge of the constructs of the universe.

After I witnessed the Creator move point of origin of the portal, I was able to channel much of the information that is in this book. I was quite pleased with the result, though I was also a little apprehensive that the negative energy might come back, but it didn't. Now positive energy pours into my cabin most of the day and night.

From this experience, I learned that vortices can be either good or bad and a portal can be connected to different places beyond this Earth. While I have known many places that have portals, moving a portal from its point of origin was new to me.

As for the negative entity that I fought with, I am sure that it will find another place or time on the planet to be.

MOVING A PORTAL

It is useful to know that it is possible to move a portal to a place that renders it harmless.

Virtues required: Adventure, bravery, faith, hope, and kindness.

Blocks: Cynicism and fear.

1. Go up to the Seventh Plane (*see pages 13 and 14*) and make the command, *'Creator of All That Is, it is commanded [or requested] that this portal is moved to a place in the universe where the energy that comes through it is wholesome.'*

2. Witness the portal being moved with the energy of kindness and love, in total confidence that it can be done. Witness the doorway being put in a place in the universe that draws positive energy into it.

3. As soon as the process is finished, rinse yourself off with Seventh-Plane energy and stay connected to it.

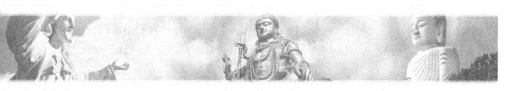

4

THE FIFTH PLANE OF EXISTENCE

As I explained in my first books, the Fifth Plane of Existence is the plane of the angels, the Council of Twelve, the soul families, the masters, and our heavenly mother and father. The masters, such as Buddha and Christ, beings who have transcended both a physical and a spiritual body, now do their work from the higher levels of the Fifth Plane.

People who channel angels and prophets and bring spirits in to perform psychic surgery and healing are connecting to this plane. Healers using this energy are, however, bound by the rules of this plane and will often heal with a sacrifice or an exchange of energy, unless they start from the Seventh Plane.

The Fifth Plane is divided into levels, which are very complicated, with many sub-divisions, but there are four main ones, each comprised of 11 degrees, making a total of 44. The 11th degree of each of the levels is the place of the Council of Twelve that rules over every soul family.

Our soul family is the group that we belonged to before we came into this incarnation. Although we incarnate into a physical family, somehow we never forget the spiritual family we left behind. Sometimes soul family members will meet one another in this incarnation and these feelings and memories will bring them together in matrimony. But this is like a brother and a sister marrying without knowing it, and because of this, there will be no lasting passion between the two people.

Soul families are now coming together to do the work of the Creator here on Earth, each guided by its Council of Twelve. Many Fifth-Plane masters who are on missions to Earth are active in these councils while living a day-to-day existence in a human body on the Third Plane. They are rising up out of their space when they are asleep to take part in the councils.

I have referred to an experience with one of these councils in my book *Advanced ThetaHealing*. When I was with this soul family council, many of the advanced beings who are here to make a difference were in that meeting with me as I begged for the chance for the Earth to be allowed to change through love. Many members of the council were voting to destroy the Earth and everyone on it through chaos, and start over. Chaos is the great destroyer.

Except for the higher degrees, the Fifth Plane is the plane of duality as a teaching tool, but this isn't the same as on the Third Plane. Duality on the Third Plane has extremes such as hot and cold, good and bad, black and white, and so on. On the lower levels of the Fifth Plane, it's more about warm and cool, good and not so good, gray and cream, and so on. On the Third Plane, we are twofold in our nature. We have good sides and bad sides, good traits and bad traits. The key is not to separate these traits but to work on the negative and become a better person. This is an aspect of the Third and Fourth Planes, but not of the higher Fifth-Plane levels. Once we reach those levels, eventually duality disappears.

Ego, too, still resides on some of the lower levels of the Fifth Plane, even though this plane is comprised of enlightened beings vibrating at different frequencies.

Energy is moved on the Fifth Plane much the same as it is on the Third Plane – with the power of thought. There, as here, virtues must be mastered in order to work with the Laws. Ultimately, the Fifth Plane is all about reaching the perfection of love.

CONNECTIONS WITH THE FIFTH PLANE

There are many prophets who have reached the Fifth Plane, such as Moses. Many have attained the sixth degree of the second level. Many of these prophets will have led good lives, but if you visit with the energy of Moses, it will be different than the energy of a master like Jesus Christ. (Both of these, I might add, were real people.) Some people connect with prophets from different times in history and many of these spiritual essences may be on some level of the Fifth Plane. But the fact that someone is mentioned in the Bible or another spiritual text doesn't mean that they are a master. Some of the prophets who are talked about in the Bible have never made it past the second level of the Fifth Plane.

I feel that you should never blindly follow anyone or any spiritual energy. The only thing to follow is the purest truth of the Creator. It's good to admire someone and listen to their wisdom, but not to the point that you become obsessed. Whenever you read a spiritual book, ask what is the truth of the content and what isn't. Be especially careful with channeled material. Anyone channeling information from the Fourth or Fifth Plane is filtering it through a Third-Plane brain that has its own beliefs. And any channeling that has a message of fear is not of the highest and best. Also, Fifth-Plane beings are incredibly developed but they are still learning themselves, so not everything they say and do is going to be entirely pure unless they are from the 33rd and 44th degrees. If you want to channel someone, you should go up to the Creator and ask for the being with the highest and best knowledge. (Of course the Creator of All That Is is above all of our concepts of gods, goddesses, heavenly fathers and heavenly mothers, not to mention all the other spirits with whom we come into contact.)

MEETING A FIFTH-PLANE BEING

This exercise will permit you to discern the different types of divinity that you may encounter in a reading. There are several levels of divinity on the Fifth Plane and each Fifth-Plane being has their own flavor and feeling.

1. Decide whom you would like to see on the Fifth Plane: an angel, god, goddess or spiritual teacher, your soul family or your Council of Twelve. Don't be surprised if you find out that you're a participant on your own council.

2. Go up to the Seventh Plane (see pages 13 and 14) and make the command: 'Creator of All That Is, It is commanded [or requested] to see and

speak with [name of spirit, god, goddess or angel], from the Fifth Plane of Existence on this [day, month, year, time]. Thank you. It is done, it is done, it is done.'

3. Visualize your consciousness being sent to the Fifth Plane.

4. Wait for the being of light to come to visit you. Speak with them.

5. When you choose to break contact, rinse yourself off in Seventh-Plane energy and stay connected to it.

Two of the highest aspects of divinity that I've experienced are the gods Shiva and Parvati. This happened when I went to India for the first time.

A Message from the Gods

The first time I went to teach in India it was as if I'd been there many times before. I've traveled to numerous places in my life, but nowhere have I felt and tasted spirituality floating in the air as it did there.

I also think that India is the land of the longest night in the world. It is as if the night lasts forever there and you become lost in time when you sleep. On one of those nights I had numerous dreams and the grand finale was when I had the same dream three times in succession. I would wake up and go right back to the same dream.

In the dream I was standing in front of the god Shiva and the goddess Parvati and I was very excited. They were emanating the most amazing divine energy. They used my sacred name and my regular name to address me, and said, 'Dearest Vianna, you are here! We welcome you. Vianna, there are many people who will like your work here, but not all of the people in India are going to be open and accept what you teach.'

I asked, 'Why not?'

They said, 'Not everyone here is ready to move forward. They haven't made it to that point yet.'

I said, 'But we all have to move forward.'

They replied, 'No, some people will not.'

'How do you deal with that?' I asked. 'It must be very frustrating.'

They said simply, 'They are what they are.'

'Why have you come to tell me this?'

With the kindest and most compassionate energy, they said, 'It is because we love them. Because they are our children and we are careful with the children of the gods. We love them all, but some of them aren't ready to change everything in their karma. Not all of them are ready to move forward, but they are all cherished by us.'

Knowing that the parental love of these deities was really important, I bowed gracefully and they left.

The weird part of the dream was that the gods and I knew one another and when they gave me this message it wasn't with a feeling of 'You can't teach in India.' In fact, they were inviting me to work with the people who *were* accepting of my teaching. They were happy that those who were ready could move their consciousness forward and release themselves from the bonds of their karma. But they needed to tell me that I had to respect those who didn't want to change.

The dream also served to remind me of the divine father and mother who watch over the children of India.

At the end of it, Guy jumped out of bed and said, 'Who's there? Is there someone in the room?'

I told him that it was only my dream and we both went back to sleep.

BEINGS OF THE FIFTH PLANE OF EXISTENCE

Angels

Warriors of Light

Archangels reside on the second level of the highest degree of the Fifth Plane. They aren't soft, cuddly, or fluffy, but are warriors of light. They go forth to protect the realms of the heavens and they take this responsibility very seriously. So they may be rather fierce.

Some healers are also warriors from the Fifth Plane. Some of us are going up in our dreams to the astral plane just to get in a fight with the forces of evil. You don't have time to fight evil all the time, though. This planet has its fair share of it and you'll constantly be in a battle of some kind. Focus on changing the people who are ready for it and don't waste your time on those who choose darkness over light.

Guardian Angels

As well as archangels, there are angels on the Fifth Plane who are sweet and kind and who minister to us, perhaps as guardians. And there are angels who have never come into contact with the Third Plane.

Guardian angels encompass a broad range of beings. They may be beings of light from the Fifth Plane, loved ones who have transcended, DNA ancestors, and animal totems. They can also manifest as fairies or nature spirits. We can have many guardian angels watching over us or only one. If we have a spiritual transition caused by a near-death experience, or any event that causes spiritual growth, new, more knowledgeable guardian angels are appointed to help us throughout our life.

Some of us have actually been angels ourselves. If you think that you were an angel before you came into a human body, you probably were. If you've been an angel in another time or place, you have inherent gifts that have not been investigated yet.

A Fourth-Plane guardian angel is different than a Fifth-Plane angel of light such as an archangel. A Fifth-Plane being of light is much more powerful. A guardian angel or guide from the Fourth Plane still has much to learn, and part of their growth process is to watch over their Third-Plane family.

I once had a reading with a woman who wanted to speak with her recently deceased husband. I went up out of my space and called him forth, but he wouldn't come. This went on for some time. Finally he came into her space and was very curt with me.

'What do you want?' he said. Then he indicated his wife. 'What does *she* want? I'm very busy!'

I told the lady I'd contacted him and she asked, 'Where is he?'

He told me, 'I'm a guardian angel for a little girl in a town in California and I'm watching over her.'

He told me the name of the town and the name of the little girl. I passed them on to the lady and she verified that this was the town in which he'd died. She later told me that the reading had motivated her to get busy in her life and become active in a hospice. Later she went to the town in California and found the little girl. To me this is validation that we're never alone – someone is always watching over us.

SENDING AN ANGEL OF PROTECTION

As an exercise in how to use Fifth-Plane energy, you can send an angel for protection and guidance to another person. If directed from the Seventh Plane, angels will simply protect the person and not become involved in the drama of good and evil.

Virtues required: Bravery, faith, forgiveness, and hope.

1. Go up to the Seventh Plane (*see pages 13 and 14*) and make the command: '*Creator, it is commanded [or requested] that a guardian angel protect [name person] from the second level of the Fifth Plane. Thank you. It is done, it is done, it is done.*'

2. Go to the Fifth Plane and witness an angel being sent to your loved one.

3. Once the angel has been sent, rinse yourself off with Seventh-Plane energy and stay connected to it.

Masters of the Fifth Plane

As spiritual essences, we are all pulsating at different frequencies. It is our ability to bend these frequencies that distinguishes the Third Plane from the Fifth Plane. The masters of the Fifth Plane are enlightened beings who have learned to bend time, matter, and subatomic particles. They can do amazing things because they have learned that their spiritual essence is not separate from the Creator. They have learned how to rejuvenate their physical, mental, emotional, and spiritual bodies.

We become a master when we reach a certain rate of vibration. If at this point we've learned all that we need to from the Third Plane of Existence, then our learning process will continue on the Fifth Plane and we can reside on one of its levels. That level is dependent on the vibration that we've attained on the Third Plane.

High masters of the Fifth Plane are composed of energy – pure energy. They have learned to control their thoughts in such a way that would make them seem gods to us. They are much more evolved than we are in our present state, but they have similarities.

High Fifth-Plane beings can become solid matter and then change back to spiritual energy. They can move through dimensions in spirit form. When angels and other otherworldly beings appear in a room and then disappear, they're traveling inter-dimensionally. When this happens, there'll be a flash of light because of the energy that's created when they make the inter-dimensional shift.

Multi-dimensional Fifth-Plane beings, known as beings of light, have learned to use the energy of pure love to create new worlds. When I talk about making a world, I'm not referring to terraforming, which is what some alien races do in order to colonize a planet, but creating whole planets, as well as the life-forms on them, spontaneously.

A master is able to create worlds on reaching the 33rd degree of the Fifth Plane. At this level, they are filled with love and understanding. They have become as Christ or Buddha. The fear of evil verses good is gone. They have mastered all the virtues and learned to bend the Laws in multi-universes with their thoughts. They are able to move life-forms back and forth between worlds in this universe and other dimensions.

For instance, my heavenly father is a high master who can bend energies and create worlds. Thirty-three beings on the 33rd degree are the beginning of the high masters who are making worlds and creating life.

The highest of the masters, however, are those of the 44th degree. When someone says (as they sometimes do) that there is an eighth plane or tenth plane, they are referring to one of the degrees of the Fifth Plane and confusing it with an essence that is beyond the Seventh Plane of Existence. But the Seventh Plane is plane of the Creator of All That Is.

Children of the Masters

Each level of the Fifth Plane holds a variety of enlightened beings. The first degree of the Fifth Plane is where the children of the masters are from.

They are nurtured on the Fourth Plane, which acts as a nursery school. Then they are sent to the First, Second, and Third Planes to grow up. Some of their parents go with them to assist them.

Children of the masters learn to filter their thoughts and acquire virtues with each lifetime on the lower planes. They learn that negative thoughts hold them back. And here on the Third Plane they learn to love. There are all kinds of love to learn, including love of a father, love of a mother and love of a friend, but first come love of God, love of self, and love of a partner. Loving one partner completely is part of the virtue of trust.

Children of the masters are learning all the time, but it should come as no surprise to learn that planet Earth isn't advancing as it should. Because of this, Fifth-Plane ascended masters have come here to teach their children to love one another.

Ascended Masters

The masters have always been watching over their children on the Third Plane. Up until 1995, however, they were only allowed to show them what to do and were never allowed to interfere directly. At this time, they were called 'the Watchers.' As they watched what their children were doing here on Earth, they perceived two possibilities for the future. One was that the Earth was ready to graduate to a more refined vibration, but it was behind schedule. The other was that it was in danger of complete collapse unless changes were made in the consciousness of their children.

So the parents of the Fifth Plane got a little worried and there was a vote among the high masters on destroying the planet and starting over or saving it from self-destruction. Some of the masters just wanted to start over and move the spirits of their children somewhere else. But other masters stood up for our world. They said, 'These are our children, our brothers and sisters! They will be devastated if we start everything over. They just need a little help. We will go and teach them if you give us a little time. If they know who they really are, they will do much better.'

It was agreed that a rescue mission of ascended masters would be sent to Earth.

However, when the rescue mission first came to Earth, they found that their vibration was so high they couldn't stay on this plane long enough to make the changes that were needed.

So a second group set off. These masters came through a spiritual portal to be born as babies and grow up in human bodies. That way, they could stay on Earth long enough to make the necessary changes. They are here now. Though they came here earlier in human history too, I've been told that there have never been as many masters here at any one time as there are now. They have come on a mission to save humanity.

What do these masters get out of this selfless action? Even a master who has come as a tutor is here to learn extra virtues. So many masters are experiencing human incarnations on Earth now that the energies of the Fifth Plane are becoming closely entwined with the Third Plane.

This second group of masters is composed of parents and older brothers and sisters of the children on Earth. To be here, they have to have reached the second or third degrees of the Fifth Plane.

These Fifth-Plane beings are still masters, even when they inhabit a Third-Plane body. This world can be difficult for them, because they have to remember who they are and why they have come here, not to mention make all the other adjustments they need to stay here. A human body vibrates at a frequency that is very different than what they are used to on the Fifth Plane. Putting a Fifth-Plane being in a human body is like taking an enormous amount of energy and putting it into a tiny bottle. It is a tight fit.

These Fifth-Plane beings carry such a high vibration that in some instances they are born sickly. The human body cannot keep up with the information of the master's mind and the vibration of their soul energy. It may take time for it to adapt. If the master is careful with the body they inhabit, sickness can be avoided. But as they grow, these children may be fighting the very DNA within them. They will always see spirits and have an instinctive connection to the Creator, and will likely feel a stranger in a strange land. They will think that the world is a cruel and merciless place and something is out of kilter in it. This is because deep within them the memories of the place they have come from are very strong.

While sleeping, they will have out-of-body experiences and accomplish goals on the Fifth Plane. This is why many healers have dreams that they are healing people and visiting with Councils of Twelve. Since Theta is a sleep wave, a ThetaHealer will use this time for what I call 'night work.' People who have experienced night work will know exactly what I'm talking about. They will remember their dreams of astral travel and will have many past-life memories. These memories and experiences may come from many different sources.

You will know you are an ascended master who is here to tutor others if you were born with the desire to help others and have the feeling that you must repeat what you have done before. This feeling might make you a little critical of yourself, so it's important not to over-analyze it. You might also think, *Surely it's a mistake that I'm here on this world. The people here are vicious and mean-spirited.* Yet you love them, and you've no idea why, because humans certainly are peculiar creatures. Nevertheless you feel bound to help them. You may even hear statements such as 'We have to save the Earth before it destroys itself' or 'The last time that we were here, we destroyed ourselves, and we've come to change the past.'

You find yourself on a mission. As a multi-dimensional being, you do 'night work' when you sleep. You want to heal the planet and encourage people to help one another. You have the ability to love, even if you weren't given love as a child. You feel obliged to awaken people.

THE AWAKENING

Many people on this planet have dim memories of a time when they were living on the Fifth Plane of Existence as masters and children of the masters. The children of the masters don't remember their experiences as clearly as the masters. They need to be awakened to their soul's potential.

I've been accused of seeing the good in people and told that my optimism concerning the human race is naïve. But if you could see people the way that I do, you'd be amazed. I see them from the perspective of their soul potential, their God-self. Once you perceive people from this perspective, you'll understand that most of us haven't even begun to realize our potential. We have no idea of what our soul has to offer the world.

For the most part, the masters who come to the Third Plane do naturally awaken to their potential. They have dreams that they are flying through space and time and memories of the amazing things they could once do.

The first thing that an awakened master does is to awaken their spiritual DNA, as in the DNA activation. A master will instinctually activate their own DNA, remember how to do healings and, at times, get discouraged by the limitations of this plane. They see what's happening in the world and they just want to go home, because on some level they know that there's a place that's much nicer than here. In the classes I teach, a recurring theme with my students is, 'I just want to go home.' This is because on a soul level they're incredibly homesick for the Fifth Plane.

The mission of the awakened masters is of course to wake up their children. If 1,000 people in every country were awakened, the course of history would be permanently changed. If only 100 people in every country were awakened, the world could be saved.

Five years ago, our chances of surviving self-destruction were only 50:50. Now I perceive that there's a 65 percent chance of succeeding. This doesn't mean that further change will be easy. I know that all kinds of bizarre things are still happening in the world. But there are positive changes too, because group consciousness is changing for the better. Only a small percentage of the planet needs to be awakened to raise the group consciousness. This awakening is the next step in our spiritual evolution on this planet.

At the present time, approximately 4 percent of the world's population are ascended masters. But the number of these masters who are consciously aware that they are masters is much lower.

Masters of the Fifth Plane come here in groups, with a leader who awakens them. Once they have awakened, they train the children of the masters. When they have trained all these children, 11 percent of the world's population will be awakened masters. As the planet progresses, so do the awakened masters.

It's easy to see the difference between a Fifth-Plane master and one of their children inhabiting a human body. This is starkly apparent in the classroom and in everyday life settings. A Fifth-Plane master will be able to listen to another person's viewpoint, while a child of a master won't be able to. A master will share their ideas and simply know truth when they see it, whereas the child of a master will sometimes be argumentative and difficult to teach. (This is one reason why there is so much plagiarizing of spiritual information.) A master, on the other hand, will always show love and respect to their teachers.

Masters cannot force their children to listen on this plane. They can only be patient and love them.

This is why we were given tools, such as the belief, feeling, and virtue work, to awaken both ascended masters and the children of the masters. This awakening will allow us to change the fate of the world. It is part of our divine timing, our mission in life – our life path.

This is why we came here. We were placed here in a third-dimensional world for a reason. It is as if someone created a video game for us, and when we play that video game, we are that character. But the larger part of us is sitting outside the video game. Our mind is focusing on it, but our soul is sitting outside it.

I remember when my granddaughter Jena was a tiny girl she believed in a higher power and believed that everything could be changed. She seemed to be watching the adults around her like a sage watching her students. But as she grew up, she began to eat the food of the Third Plane both physically and consciously. Also, her hormones began to kick in, and when this happens to a young person, they can lose sight of their past experiences and spiritual power for a while. Some people reawaken later in life and claim their powers of the spirit. The most prevalent awakening years seem to be 27, 31, 34, 37, 41, and 42. Other people don't have to be awakened at all – they know who they are throughout their lives.

Many young people these days are drawn to drugs and alcohol because they are too psychic and want to be able to turn it off. This is why it is so important to teach a gifted child to control their psychic abilities. With proper training, these young people can avoid this dangerous time and will never have this problem again.

We were all put here to learn, and the way we learn is through duality. We learn to love. We learn to overcome fear. We learn all the raw emotions. We learn to make the right choices. We learn that with free agency as our guide we can focus our thoughts, acquire virtues, and work with the Laws. Once we start doing this, we graduate from school.

Technically, we have to learn to stop killing each other. This would be a nice change. The Earth was supposed to be more evolved by now.

Fifth-Plane Soul, Third-Plane Body

Once you realize that you're a Fifth-Plane being, your soul may find that it wants to go back to where the energy is more compatible with it. Many of us are in a constant battle between staying here and going home. But the truth is, instead we can achieve a level of mastery where we don't have to get old or die and we can move back and forth between the Third and Fifth Planes of Existence.

The way to do this is through undertaking three kundalini openings without dying from the experience. Then when we return home to the Fifth Plane, we'll go to a higher place.

The Kundalini Openings

- The first kundalini opening is at the base of the spine.

  This opening is the *awakening*. It opens a person to their psychic abilities. Many people become overwhelmed if it happens too quickly. This is why it should take place in a Theta state. You can do this through the meditation to the Seventh Plane. This will help it to happen gradually. The DNA activation can help this process.

- The second kundalini opening begins in the heart.

  With this opening, a person knows true unconditional love and has the ability to overcome sorrow. After this, they are able to change the lives of others.

- The third and last opening is at the crown, in the pineal gland.

  This gives a person a pure essence that changes their aura color to white. With this opening, they realize that they are living in an illusion and can create consciously with pure thought.

  In the past this opening meant that the person no longer wished to sustain a third-dimensional body and had made the choice to die in order to ascend to the Fifth Plane. They had acquired all the virtues and there was no need to continue the game of life. However, it's now possible to stay in the game if you wish to.

YOUR FIFTH-PLANE SACRED NAME

On the Fifth Plane you have one specific vibration. So your Fifth-Plane sacred name encompasses your whole being and holds the highest aspect of your soul energy.

Knowing it enables you to perform healings more effectively. For instance, I say to the Creator; 'Creator, this is Vianna [plus my sacred name] and I would like a healing on this person.'

Remember, your Fifth-Plane sacred name isn't a past-life name – I can guarantee it isn't something like 'Cleopatra' or 'Julius Caesar.' These are very popular past-life names, and so is 'Jesus.' When people come up and tell me that they were Jesus Christ in a past life, I ask them if they used to live in Mexico or another Latin country where people love to name their children Jesus. I ask them, 'Which Jesus were you?'

Don't get me wrong; it may be that someone is genetically related to the one and only Jesus Christ (he did have brothers and sisters, and possibly children). This may explain the memories and feelings they are having. There may be many reasons why they are having these experiences.

One may be that when you love people unconditionally, you love them with your higher self, and this means you reach the rank of Christ, i.e., you are totally connected to God. And when you reach a certain level on the Fifth Plane and you are a mother who loves your children unconditionally, you reach the rank of Mary. But these names won't be your sacred name. To discover that, go up and ask the Creator.

YOUR FIFTH-PLANE SACRED NAME

What is your sacred name on the Fifth Plane of Existence?

1. Go up to the Seventh Plane (see pages 13 and 14) and make the command: 'Creator of All That Is, It is commanded [or requested] that I know my sacred name from the Fifth Plane of Existence. Thank you. It is done, it is done, it is done.'

2. Visualize your consciousness being sent to the Fifth Plane.

3. Wait for the vibration of your sacred name to come to you.

4. Once you choose to break contact, disconnect by rinsing yourself off in Seventh-Plane energy and stay connected to it.

TIME AND SPACE
Space Travel on the Wings of Thought

There are fourth and fifth-dimensional worlds with civilizations that have learned how to move through time, space, and dimensions. There are also third-dimensional races that have learned how to travel over vast distances by folding space. In our own future, just as on these worlds, space travel is going to be done by bending time.

But a far more advanced mode of space travel is sending focused thought. The human mind is unbelievably expansive and has abilities we still don't fully understand. Once we do understand the full extent of our capabilities, our mind will integrate fully with our soul and we will be able to move through the universe without mechanical aids.

To better explain this concept, we can say that the *spirit* is in the body but the *soul* is multi-dimensional and is able to travel vast distances and experience infinite experiences. Our soul energy is the energy that exists after death, and this means that it becomes Fifth-Plane energy. However, when a Fifth-Plane being travels back and forth between dimensions, it takes a great deal of energy. That's why a Fifth-Plane being appears surrounded by luminescent energy.

This kind of theory is out of many people's comfort zone. When faced with it, many of my students will respond with disbelief, anger, or fear. I believe that these feelings are partly created to keep us locked into our situations here. What if you could focus your thoughts and immediately access a Law of the universe to create instant change? What if you could remember how to bend time as an ascended master?

Time and the Ascended Master

In the co-creative process of ThetaHealing, time doesn't exist. This is because thought can move faster than the speed of light and in doing so it can bend the time–space continuum. Every time you send out your consciousness to the planes of existence you're performing an act of Theta brainwave dimensional time travel.

Since you're an inter-dimensional being having a third-dimensional experience and there's no such thing as time, what makes you think that this life is the only experience that you're having? Perhaps you're living several lives at once at different times in history, or even in different times or places in the universe.

For instance, I know I'm in a human body, but I can put myself in a state of mind so that I can experience one of my past lives in great detail. The next realization is the awareness that my soul is in other times and places, having multiple life experiences. I come to this realization by connecting to these multiple lives and maintaining this state of mind. Then I can be consciously aware of them.

Bending the Law of Time

When we influence the Law of Time, remember we're only *bending* it. We don't change it for the whole planet, only for our little world. Let's say that there are two of us starting out for work in the morning in different cars using the same route. If I bend time to get to work, it may take me 38 minutes, but the other person may take 45 minutes. I'm bending time for myself but not for anyone else. I'm sharing this planet with billions of other souls who have free agency and I'm not allowed to break the imperative of an Ultimate Truth. Remember, the best ways to lose your gifts of healing are to start denying there's a God and interfering with another person's free agency.

When we've acquired the ability to bend time on a spiritual level, we can 'phase shift' into the past to create a new 'present' and thereby change the future. I believe that part of me is in the future watching what I'm doing now. I know this because I can remember things happening before they happen.

If we can validate that something is going to happen before it does, this also validates that our spirit goes back and forth through the realms of present, past, and future to create the future.

People ask me, 'How can the past and the future be happening at once when I'm living in the now? How can I still see the future and the past? How does that work?'

My answer to this is two questions: 'How can you tell people that they'll get well unless you're seeing them getting well in the future? How can you do a healing if you don't think you can affect the future?'

When we tell someone's body to get better (and obviously this is an outcome they want), I propose we create our own reality and to an extent we can see it before it happens.

Predictions of the Future

When we see into the future, however, are our fears creating what we see or are we making a prediction free from fear and our own beliefs? There's a big difference. For instance, I've watched a friend of mine actually create a situation so that her husband eventually left her. I think that her fears were so strong that she manifested the situation into reality. I think that this is the same with soul mates. Many of us have such a fear of never meeting our soul mate that we never do.

In the end, it doesn't matter if what happens is a prediction or a manifestation, as long as the outcome is beneficial. However, there are situations where knowing the difference between the two can be helpful. What's important is to believe that the future isn't set and can be changed. It's also good to be aware that you may be stopping yourself from seeing and creating your own future because of the acceptance of this fear from others, as in the following story.

I once met a young woman who wanted to have children. She visited a psychic and asked about it and was told that she would never have any. When she came to me for a reading, I said to her, 'Now that's really funny, because I see you with three children in the future.'

She said, 'Oh no, I physically can't have children.'

Time went past and I saw her again. She told me she now had three children.

Apparently the psychic had seen her worst fear and projected it in the reading as true information. This is the difference between a reading from the third eye and going to the crown and beyond to the Seventh Plane of Existence.

Reading the Future and Remembering the Future

In ThetaHealing we teach two ways to see the future: reading the future and remembering the future.

Reading the future is simply perceiving the most likely future. On the surface, we are all creating our own future with our thoughts and actions. Each one of us is weaving a pattern, a mosaic that represents our life. These actions can be changed by free will. With most people, however, their future is predictable because they don't know how to change the lifestyles and patterns that keep them bound by what some people call 'fate.'

But once a person has the realization that they're not bound by fate, there are usually many outcomes in their future. Life has infinite possibilities and the future can always be changed by small actions done at the right time and in the right way. This puts responsibility for the future into the hands of the individual.

A good reader can predict the most likely outcome as it relates to someone's future, but the power of individual free will can bend fate and time within the beauty that is divine timing, the soul's mission in this life.

The following story tells how I came to some of these realizations.

The night before I was traveling home from a class in New Zealand I suddenly had the feeling that I should go up and check to see how the trip was going to unfold in the near future. I saw that we were going to be delayed for some reason and that I would have to stay the night in Salt Lake City and wouldn't have a change of clothes.

At this point, I asked myself, *Did I create this delay in some way?* I thought that perhaps in the act of visualizing that I'd be delayed I was somehow creating it. However, I packed an extra set of clothes in my carry-on just in case.

When you've traveled for a while, you realize that once you set off, you're in the capable hands of the airlines. No matter what, you're going to get to your destination. It may not be on the day you wanted, but you will get there. In addition, you will get your checked luggage ... eventually.

When you're traveling on multiple flights, it seems that your carry-on luggage gets heavier and heavier as you go. Because of this, I don't put a lot in my carry-on. If you travel as much as I do, you learn what you can live without and what you cannot. So as I was packing the extra clothes, Guy asked me what I was doing.

I told him, 'We're going to get delayed and I'm packing clothes just in case.'

Tired from the long trip, he said, 'Okay, whatever. You can pack them if you want to, but we're leaving really early tomorrow morning and I hope we're not going to be delayed. Are you sure you're not creating this?'

I said, 'No, I don't think so.'

From the very first flight out of New Zealand, we were delayed. Our flight out of Los Angeles to Salt Lake was also delayed and we ended up sleeping in the airport for a few hours. When we finally got to Salt Lake City we'd missed all the flights out for that night and were told we'd have to spend the night there. The airline put us up in a nice hotel and guess who had a change of clothes? Believe me, at this point on the trip, clean clothes were a wonderful luxury!

Obviously, I'd changed my future by packing an extra set of clothes, but I hadn't felt that I could change the planes being delayed.

Some weeks later, I began to have a funny feeling about the next return trip I was due to make, this time from Italy. I went up out of my space and asked to remember my future on this trip. I remembered that we were delayed in Washington, DC, and had to stay overnight in Virginia. This didn't make any sense to me. Why would I have to stay overnight in

Virginia if I was in Washington, DC? Still, I saw that I needed a change of clothes, so yet again I packed extra in my carry-on.

This time when Guy saw what I was doing, he said, 'Hmm, I think I'll pack a change of clothes too.'

Sure enough, the weather delayed us and we were stuck in Washington, DC. All the planes were grounded and the closest hotel we could stay in was in Virginia, an hour away by taxi. Since the thought of sleeping on the floor of the airport was a little more than we could bear, we slept in the taxi until we arrived at the hotel.

So I ask you, could I have prevented all this? No, I'm sorry, but I couldn't stop those thousands of people being delayed that night with the strength of my subconscious mind. However, I saw the circumstances that could be changed within my own paradigm, and I changed them.

Here's how it works: you can't *see* your future because it hasn't happened yet, but you can *remember* your future because everything's happening simultaneously. So you go up and ask the Creator of All That Is to show you something specific, saying, 'The last time I did this, what happened?'

This concept can make some people panicky, because they don't want to see their future. If you feel panicky, it's time to do belief work on any issues about the future.

BELIEF WORK ON THE FUTURE

Energy test for:

'It's wrong to see what I'm creating now.'

'Every decision I make can make a positive change in my future.'

'I create my own reality.'

Download:

'I know what it *feels like* and I know *how* to live my day-to-day life without being nervous or fearful about the future.'

'I know how to practice healing without getting discouraged.'

'I have the patience with myself to attain mastership.'

─────────────────

Some people panic because of death doors. But if one is coming up for them, does that mean they have to take it? No, they have the choice, and I tell them this. For instance, if I'm doing a reading with somebody and see that they have a death door in a couple weeks, I may say, 'You know, you have to make some decisions if you want to stay here on this planet.'

Decisions are the key to change. The personal decisions you make affect your future. When you go up and remember your own future, you're looking for how to change things by making different decisions on a personal level.

There are times when you look at your future and you can't see very far ahead because you haven't created it yet. But it isn't wrong to see what you're creating now so that you can change it. Remembering the future is effective when it comes to changing world events through small acts of courage.

There's an old wives' tale that says that an intuitive can't see into their own future. This isn't true. Not only can they see their future, they can create it as well.

In one narrow, mechanistic view of reality, it's said that you can't see your future because it simply hasn't happened yet. But I believe that the past, present, and future are the same thing, and that they don't exist independently of one other. I believe that we live in all three at once, and just as we can remember our past, we can also remember our future. Our DNA lineage is a chain connecting the past with the present and the present with the future. I think that there is a part of our consciousness that is beyond past, present, and future, and this is the God-self, the spark of creation that is within all of us and allows us to change reality.

If you connect to the Creator and ask to *remember* the future, you can see it crystal clear. This admittedly takes practice. In many instances, people try to see – or create – the future they want, without considering those around them and their own divine timing, the plan they agreed on for this life. A good example of this is when people think that they can throw spells (throwing thoughts at another person in order to hurt them or to control their life). This is a Fifth-Plane action and goes against the Law of Free Agency.

A good intuitive is always impervious to negative thoughts of others and can easily realize that they are creating everything in their life and, in doing so, become aware of the lives and rights of others.

There are several ways to remember your future. One way is to go up to the Creator and ask to read the Akashic Records. But I prefer to go up to the Creator and stand at the edge of the universe, where you can see your past, present, and future at the same time. This has one added advantage: once you can see your future, you can simply change it – or better yet, create it within the enormity of your divine timing.

REMEMBERING YOUR FUTURE

1. Go up to the Seventh Plane of Existence (see pages 13 and 14) and make the command: 'Creator of All That Is, it is commanded [or requested] that I see and remember my future now. Thank you. It is done, it is done, it is done.' This will take you to the Sixth Plane of Existence on the outer edge of the universe. This is where the Law of Cause and Effect resides and where you can see what your actions have created in your life up to this point, both future and past.

2. Stand there for a moment. It will appear as if there are two mirrors, one on either side of you, and you can see all the past and all the future in them.

3. You can also command to go to the Akashic Records via the Law of Cause and Effect, which overlaps the Law of Time, which overlaps the Akashic Records. Be present there and see what you are creating in your life.

4. As you look at your future, say, 'The last time this happened, what did I do next to make things better?'

The most effective (and my favorite) way to remember the future is the following:

1. Go up to the Seventh Plane and command to be taken to a day after the event that you're asking about.

2. Witness your consciousness in that time.

3. Make the command: *'Creator, the last time that this event happened, what happened?'* or *'Creator, I can remember what happened.'*

4. Observe silently.

5. When you've finished seeing the future, bring yourself back to the present time.

6. When the event that you remembered comes into the present, check to see how much you were able to perceive. Don't dwell on how much you got wrong, but on what you got right. That way, you'll train your brain to perceive the right future.

When you first do this exercise, you may focus too much on your fears, thus getting the wrong answers or creating negative energy in your future. Counter this with belief work.

It's best only to go a couple of days into the future at first.

If you go forward one year to look at the future, you may realize that there's more than one significant event in store for you. When you look this far at the future, you may want to break it down by the months of the year and ask to see all the significant events in each one. You may also want to focus on the different aspects that life has to offer, such as the home, work, relationships, and so on.

You may feel a little dizzy when you come back after going this far into the future and it's best to ground yourself in the current time and place. You're training your mind to do something that it may not be used to. So don't be discouraged if you see something happening in January and it doesn't happen until February. You got it right, but the timing was a bit off. It is all about getting the right information and not torturing yourself for getting the wrong information. Looking into the future requires practice, practice, and more practice. But don't practice so much that you're constantly looking at the future without enjoying the present.

When I do future readings, I look to see if it is spring, summer, fall, or winter when an event is happening. This may be difficult for people who live in a place that doesn't have distinct seasons. Also, if you're looking at events in the southern hemisphere, remember that the seasons are the opposite way round.

REMEMBERING THE FUTURE FOR ANOTHER PERSON

In this exercise you will remember the future for another person. It's best to remember only a week ahead and not attempt to change events months from the present. Before using this exercise in a serious situation, you must have already seen the future correctly at least 100 times.

1. Ask the person what they want to know about an upcoming event in the future.

2. Ask their permission to remember their future.

3. Go up to the Seventh Plane (*see pages 13 and 14*) and make the command: *'Creator of All That Is, it is commanded [or requested] that I see and remember [name person]'s future now. Thank you. It is done, it is done, it is done.'*

4. The Creator will take you up to the Law of Cause and Effect. Silently observe. See what the person is creating in their life.

5. Ask, 'The last time this happened, what can [person] do to make things better?'

FATE-CHANGERS

As beings who have been sent here to help the Earth in its ascent toward love and peace, ascended masters have the ability to do something that I call the 'do-over.' In fact many of us have come back to change events in our lives that we weren't able to change the first time that we came here.

We do this through our future selves, who are conscious that the past needs to be changed in order to accomplish our mission in the future.

Up until 1995, ascended masters weren't allowed to interfere with the Earth's future, but now they can take action to prevent futures that happened before. By 'before' I mean that there's a very strong possibility that there's one future where the world comes to an end. Prophets have predicted apocalyptic events and I think that there are spiritual energies that have come back to change the events leading up to this disaster.

Not only can an ascended master perceive the most logical future, they can also see what will happen if different decisions are made. This means that they can see multiple possible futures. They have the ability to see multiple futures from just one event, and the most likely outcomes. If they use the 'remember the future' technique, they can see the overall outcome on a grand scale as it relates to the Earth. By remembering the future in this way, it's possible for them to change events such as massacres, social uprisings, war, and other violent acts.

I call the people who use this technique, on whatever level, 'fate-changers,' because they remember what happened last time and change the future by recognizing what needs to be changed now. They also see their decisions in the future and make changes there too. I believe that there are so many fate-changers on Earth at this time that two realities are overlapping: 'the end of the world' and 'the new beginning for the world.'

The more we make choices that create positive outcomes, the more likely it is that we won't bring about our own demise. People who are involved in healing in particular will carry out small acts of kindness that will result in powerful changes that can save the world.

As fate-changers, we have a list of things we came here to alter and a list of people we came here to help, and we're not going to give up until these things are done. Even if we don't complete these lists in this lifetime, we can come back to the context of this lifetime to complete what we came to do. I believe that we come back several times to the same time and space in different attempts to change a situation.

I believe that our soul has an expansive energy. The soul-intelligence is amazing in that it's far more than this Third-Plane body. This means that it can be in many places at once.

Changing fate is the difference between going against the current of Third-Plane consciousness and being the dead fish that flows down the river. My job, and the job of others like me, is to offer the awakening so that people can change their beliefs and make the life that they want for themselves. When I first met Guy, I told him that we were here for a special reason. Our spirits came to this time and place for a specific mission.

If something isn't done now, the self-destructive nature of humanity will win out, as it has done in many possible futures. But we're learning we can make a difference by healing the collective consciousness. The more we come to the spiritual realization that we have something important to do, the more we'll also come to the next realization: that we're more than this body, more than this space and time.

Déjà Vu

Have you ever wished you'd taken the advice of an old friend and done something the way they'd suggested? Have you ever made a decision and wished that you had it to do over again? These *déjà vu* 'do-over' messages are the Creator whispering to our soul.

I believe that a *déjà vu* experience occurs when we're getting close to an important event that needs to be changed. Our future selves are becoming aware of being in this space and time and that the time is coming to change this event.

What if you knew that there was a future self and we were here to change things? What if you knew when, how, and where to change things? What we do and what we say in this world are so important, because we're here to get it right. Once we get it right in this space and time, our future self will no longer have to come back to change events in the past.

What if a decision you make this morning affects the rest of the world? What if you tell one person that they can change the planet and they go on and become the president of a country, all because you said that they could do it?

There was a time a few years ago when I was having difficult situations in my life. When I looked at my life from the perspective of the soul, I saw that the things I'd done this time were much better than the things I'd done the last time I lived this life. The last time, things had got very out of hand, but this time they'd been handled in a better way because I hadn't overreacted. At first I'd wanted to react negatively, but I'd been able to listen to the advice I'd received from the divine. This is why it's important to know when you're in a 'do-over' moment.

To me, the feeling of *déjà vu* is a warning sign that an event is coming in my life that needs to be changed and my soul-self is reminding me to step up to the challenge. When I have a *déjà vu* experience, I say to myself, 'What did I do the last time this happened? This time I'm going to do it differently.'

I believe that every time you have a *déjà vu* experience, it's because you've lived this life before and you now have the opportunity to make changes in it. *Déjà vu* is an early warning system for upcoming events that need to be changed.

Saving a Life

This story is an example of how to use a message from the future to change what happened the last time that you lived this life.

Let me give you some background: Guy has an ex-wife and, like many *divorcés*, the only contact they have now is through the children they had when they were together. Through Guy's son Tyrel we knew that his ex-wife was in a relationship with a big and very volatile woman and the two of them got into violent fights.

One afternoon I was at home minding my own business, sitting on the couch watching television with Guy. Then, without thinking about what I was saying, I looked over at Guy and said, 'Tonight is the night that your ex-wife gets killed.'

Guy looked at me for a few seconds and said, 'What?!'

I said, 'Her girlfriend shoots her tonight.'

Incredulous, Guy asked, 'What are you talking about?!'

'*The last time this happened*,' I told him, 'she got shot and killed.'

'What can I do about it?'

Without asking me any more questions, Guy immediately went to call Tyrel, who was living with his mother at the time.

'What are you doing tonight?' he asked.

Tyrel said, 'I'm leaving the house. Those two are fighting again.'

Guy said, 'Tyrel, do me a favor – don't go anywhere tonight. Stay at home and keep an eye on things. Just as a favor. Okay?'

'Okay, Dad.'

A half-hour later, Tyrel called us back. It seems the fight had escalated. The girlfriend had pulled a gun on his mother with the intention of shooting her.

Because of my warning and Guy's intervention, Tyrel was there, watchful and ready. He was able to wrestle the big woman to the ground and courageously disarm her. He likely saved his mother's life.

After that, the police became involved and that put a definite end to the relationship. The woman stalked Tyrel's mother for some time until finally the police arrested her on another charge and she was jailed.

If it hadn't been for my message from the future, matters would have taken quite another course and I think that Guy's ex-wife would have been killed that night. We were given the opportunity to change the outcome and do the right thing. I changed the future because I perceived what had happened the last time it had happened. That perception came with a *déjà vu* feeling to it – it was as if it was one of the things that I'd come back from the future to change.

This experience not only saved someone's life but also helped Guy and me to develop virtues, because both of us overcame our resentment for someone who had been difficult in the past.

Moments of *déjà vu* aren't only indicators of small events but can also tell us when we have the opportunity to change the outcome of large events such as hurricanes, wars, and earthquakes. If we practice going up to the Creator and asking to remember 'what happened the last time,' the situation can be corrected by making a different choice at the right time.

FUTURE WORK FOR THE FATE-CHANGER

To change the future:

1. Connect to the Seventh Plane of Existence (*see pages 13 and 14*) and go forward in time to a day after the event that you wish to remember.

2. If the outcome isn't desirable, come back to the present and change the decisions that will change the future.

3. Then go into the future to see if these decisions have changed the outcome.

4. Download from the Creator: *'I know how to create my future by going back in the past and influencing the present to influence the future.'*

Like anything else, this takes practice and it may be that not everything will be changed this time around.

I'm unsure as to how many lifetimes we get to 'do over.' But I am sure that we're here to make a difference to this planet. We're here to teach the right way – the way of love. All we need to make this transformation of consciousness on this planet is to have 100 ThetaHealing teachers change their beliefs and offer the possibility of awakening to every country. Could you imagine what 1,000 teachers could do? If there were 10,000 healers of *any* modality that embraced love, we could change what happened the last time we were here.

The Walk-in

Many years ago I experimented with hypnosis. In one of the sessions, I made the statement that I'd only been in a human body a few times but I'd been a walk-in 274 times. At the time, I didn't consciously know what the term 'walk-in' meant, but under hypnosis, I somehow did. As time went on, I learned more about what it meant to me.

Hindus believe that a walk-in is an advanced spirit who hasn't finished what they needed to do in their life and comes back as a spiritual essence from another dimension to make certain that things happen as they should. It takes over the body of a person who is going to die or wants to die to complete their mission. This doesn't mean that the spirit that takes over the body is a wayward spirit or that the person is possessed – a walk-in spirit is an enlightened being who has come on a mission of goodness and has made an agreement on a soul level with the person who is leaving their body.

I believe that many of us are here to complete our divine timing, our mission in this life. And if we don't accomplish all that we came to here to do, we can either come back and use the body of someone who isn't using it any longer, or, when our spirit is leaving our body, an enlightened spirit can walk into it to finish our mission. This can explain the personality changes that some people have when they have a near-death experience.

In other instances a walk-in is inside us living as a spiritual essence, sharing our physical body with us through an *agreement*. The body is animated by the energy of the extra spirit. This is different than a soul experiencing multiple lives at one time.

However, walk-ins are rarer than you might think. Many people who are psychically aware have the strong feeling that they have 'jumped' into their own life, but I feel that in most instances they are confusing a walk-in with their own energetic self that has come back from the future to change something.

I also believe that what people call a walk-in can actually be part of their higher self that has come from a past life or a future life. And when someone integrates more of their present higher self into their body, they may think it's a walk-in too.

Some people shut down their psychic abilities when they are children and then, when these abilities are awakened later in life, they think that another spirit has walked into their body. That somehow explains the great change that is happening to them.

All these people would categorize themselves as walk-ins, but they haven't had a spirit take over their body at all. All that's happened is that they've come to realize their spiritual qualities and psychic abilities. This may make them very different from their family. Sometimes they may prefer to think of themselves as walk-ins rather than attempt to explain themselves to others – or even themselves.

When someone comes to me and tells me they're a walk-in, I teach them what it feels like for their soul to be safe in their body. This helps to integrate the soul and the body so that there's no separation.

DIVINE TIMING

Many years ago when I first started to do readings, I met a man in Idaho Falls who was also into alternative healing and taught NLP. We used to have conversations about the meaning of life and why we were here. One day, he asked me what I wanted to accomplish in life. My answer perplexed him. I told him, 'I want to see someone's arm grow back.'

He told me that such a thing was impossible and this was an unrealistic goal to have. As our conversation continued, he said, 'Vianna, there's something wrong with you. You keep thinking that you're going to save the planet. In reality, this thinking is an illusion. People must save themselves and you should pay attention to yourself. Don't pay attention to the rest of the world.'

Inwardly, I felt that he was selfish in his thinking. I knew that one person *could* make a difference. I also knew that there had to be more people like me out there in the world, people who were part of my soul family, people who wanted the world to stop acting stupid. Then I began to have visions of groups of people making a difference in the world.

These early visions of soul families coming together are part of the reason why ThetaHealing is the way it is. We aren't a hierarchy. We don't have generals or captains. We're all in a particular state of mind that has the premise of 'we can make a difference.' We're a soul family on this plane because that is what we were on the Fifth Plane, the place we came from. We work together because we love one another. This is the only way that ThetaHealing can spread out. It doesn't mean that everyone has to be part of ThetaHealing. All that needs to be done is to create a tipping point in group consciousness that will create change in millions of people. It may be that all that is needed is for people to change a few beliefs. This alone may be enough to tip the balance of the world toward goodness.

Creating ThetaHealing was actually the second stage of my divine timing. Divine timing is what we agreed and planned to do in this existence. When our soul awakens to its divine purpose, the time to fulfill it has come. When this happens, the divine timing door opens and we're given an opportunity to carry out our mission.

How we do that is up to us. But our soul will make sure we're where we're supposed to be to accomplish our divine timing. This is because the needs of the soul outweigh the conscious mind in importance.

The first stage of my divine timing was having my children. An astrologer once told me that my family came down with me for a divine purpose. This could be true, since they all work for me. They were the first members of my soul family on this plane. ThetaHealing is the gathering of the rest of my soul family.

I know I have four major divine timings. The third is to finish certain paintings that I saw myself creating when I was a teenager. When I finally saw my fourth, it stressed me out because I'm still working on my divine timing number two. ThetaHealing is a very extensive divine timing!

In one of my classes, a student once asked me, 'Isn't it hard to stand up all day and teach ThetaHealing when you know that most of the world doesn't believe in it? When they think that you're teaching something weird?'

I said to her, 'What are you talking about? *They* are the weird ones, not me! I'm the one who's *normal!*'

This is why I teach ThetaHealing. I believe in it and I'm awakening my soul family. I teach believers and I really don't care what other people think. It doesn't take much courage to teach people what I believe to be the truth, but it isn't always easy. There are times when I'm bone-tired but I still get up to do readings for people who need me. There's something inside me that compels me help people.

In the early years of teaching there were times when I'd be worn down from travel and would get a cold the day before a class. Guy would say, 'You should cancel the class. You aren't feeling well and you can't teach like this.'

But I'd tell him, 'No, I'm teaching.'

Then, right before I had to teach, I'd recover.

Guy thought this was weird, and of course to some it might seem strange. But I can do this because there's something inside me that pushes me forward. Something that says, 'This planet can be changed.'

The drive that I have to teach has to do with my divine timing. And as time went on, Guy began to understand that no matter what challenges this life had in store for us, no matter what the odds, our divine timing had to be accomplished.

I've learned that it's important to distinguish between divine timing and your own beliefs. For years, I was afraid that I would die on Guy. But in truth, it was *his* fear that I would die on him and nothing to do with a set future event. It was his fear, not the divine river, that was talking to me.

However, I did know, on some weird level, that if I ever went into a coma, I'd be coming back to life. I believe that the little coma incident that happened to me in Rome in 2007 was somehow in my divine plan. At some level, I had to come as close to death as I could and come back to life. I think that I brought myself back from the point of death because I'd designed it that way. I think that it was one of the most important experiences that I set up for myself. A month before the coma, I told everybody that I wasn't going to teach DNA 3 (one of the ThetaHealing courses) until I'd gone into a coma or I'd brought someone back from the dead. Obviously, I was pushing for that experience on some level, to see if it could be done.

In ancient times, that was the test: 'Are you good enough to die and come back?' When I came back, I felt very secure and ready to say, 'I've lived this. I know this. I know you can go there and come back. I know you can heal your body.' Maybe this isn't something we all ought to experience, but I know it was part of my divine timing. I told Guy when I married him, 'If I go into a coma, don't worry, I'm coming back. Don't turn the life support machine off – I'm coming back.'

As a child, I had a fear of institutions. I had visions of being tied up and locked in a room where no one could hear me. In the hospital in Rome, I was tied down because they were giving me so much prednisone that if I'd stood up, my heart would have exploded. And the Italian doctors couldn't understand what I was saying and I sure couldn't understand them. They just stood there in confusion when I tried to speak to them. In the end they had to get doctors who could understand English. And then flashes from my childhood came back. I'd seen all this before!

Since then I've seen many visions of alternative realities and alternative futures. I've seen hectic scenes of Earth changes. I've seen the destruction of the Earth. I've come to understand that the possibility of that particular future can change from day to day. If you go up and ask, 'Is the Earth going to be destroyed?' you're going to get a different answer every day, because we change our *beliefs* every day.

What would you think if you knew that your divine timing was to help 224,000 people? It might be overwhelming to know this. What would you think if you knew you were going to change the lives of 1,400,042 people through your very existence? You might be too overwhelmed to follow through with your mission.

But if your diving timing is to be in Singapore on May 18, 2018, to help a particular person, you're going to be there to help that person. Your divine timing might be something as small as saying the right word at the right time in the right place to inspire someone, and this act will change the vibration of the world.

You may not believe me, but it doesn't matter. That's why I don't tell people their divine timing. I let them find it out for themselves.

The Japanese Tsunami

Though I don't tell people their divine timing, when I'm teaching there are times when I get little flashes of my students' divine timing. These visions can make me uncomfortable, particularly when I know that I can't do anything to change the outcome. Acceptance can be a very difficult thing.

The year before the 2011 Japanese earthquake and tsunami I did a teaching seminar in Japan. During one of the classes, I began to see parts of the students' divine timing. I had a vision of one lady in the front row teaching thousands of people in an auditorium. Then I looked at the lady next to her and I was shocked by what I saw: she was being covered over with water and was being pulled away by it. As she was being pulled away, she pushed a baby up to the shore where it would be safe and then she was gone. This vision really upset me.

The next time I was in Japan was two weeks after the tsunami. The first person I looked for in my class was that woman. I knew she wasn't going to be there, but I looked anyway. She wasn't there. This made me very sad. From that time onward, I didn't want to look at people's divine timing.

Then the Creator told me, 'Vianna, some people live their whole life to carry out a single divine act. If that woman's last divine timing was to save a very important baby, that was an amazing way to go to the next life.'

I don't know how old the baby that was saved would be now, but I can tell you one thing: he's going to be an amazing soul!

Not all divine timings are going to have a happy outcome, but I guess it depends on how you look at it.

Divine Timing is Immutable

What I can say is when we live our life in harmony with our divine timing, life is easier. Divine timing is always amazing. There is the sparkle of a miracle about it. It's always for our highest and best, even if we don't fully understand it. Some people seem to think it's like a rule, and rules are made to be broken. This is far from the truth. Divine timing simply is an immutable quintessence, like the sun rising each day.

Sometimes I hear people say, 'I'm going to change my divine timing.' If you want to attempt that, fine. You'll simply recreate it and the same thing will happen anyway.

Other people say, 'I don't want to carry out my divine timing. I want to create my own life.' Okay, whatever. If it makes you happy to think this, fine. In the end, you'll probably end up carrying out your divine timing anyway, probably without knowing that you are.

Others say; 'Okay, I'm ready. I know what I'm here for and I want to get it over with.'

Like *you* want to get it over with!

Yet others say, 'I don't believe in divine timing.'

I tell them, 'That doesn't matter. It's going to happen anyway.'

It doesn't matter what kind of tantrum you throw here on Earth, you'll still be guided to your divine timing.

I once had a friend who said that they could pull and cancel a person's divine timing if they didn't want to do it. I found this to be amusing because I know that the minute you go to sleep, your soul recreates your divine timing because your soul knows what you really need to do.

Remember, you came here because you wanted to. It may not seem that way on the surface, but on a soul level, you came here to make a difference. Now you're learning how to do it.

If the path to your divine timing becomes difficult, it may be time to discuss things with the Creator. But if you go up and say, 'Creator, this path isn't very comfortable for me, may I choose not to do this?', what sort of answer do you think you're going to receive? That's right, compassionate laughter. (God has a very good sense of humor.)

Then you may hear this answer: 'My child, the path to your divine timing isn't always going to be easy. It may be difficult for a time, but then all of a sudden everything will fall into place and things will work for you. When they do, it means that your divine timing is working for you and you aren't working against it. In the meantime, it may be time to change your beliefs.'

In order to be prepared for our divine timing we must also clear our blocks surrounding such simple things as money. Are you prepared to receive all the abundance that the Creator has to give you? The Creator's unconditional love energy brings love, laughter, family, friends, and plenty of abundance for those who use it, for the Creator is not poor, the Creator is omnipotent. When we begin to use our birthright we'll not only bring abundance to our own life, we'll bring it to those around us as well.

The one thing I emphasize is the question: 'How do you want to reach your divine timing?' For instance, would you like to be a millionaire or just be scraping by? Since we're all going to arrive at our divine timing destination, it is important that we pick the right road to get there. That road can be anything we choose it to be.

I feel that I've tried to escape this world several times, but because of my divine timing, I've been brought back from the brink of death to finish what I was sent here to do. I can remember lying on a bed in the hospital with my blood pressure bottoming out. I can remember my spirit starting to leave my body and these little voices telling me, 'Oh no, not yet, Vianna. You're not dying now. You're going to live.' This happened to me enough times that I decided that I was going to have fun while I was here, because leaving wasn't an option, at least not yet.

With divine timing, more can be accomplished than you might imagine. And if we can see our future accurately, we can always *improve upon* our divine timing. It has been my experience that there are only two things that cannot be changed: babies who are going to be born and soul mates who are going to find each other.

Perceiving Your Divine Timing

Your divine timing is unique to you. Other people can perceive parts of it, but only you can see all of it. The Creator will show it to you when you're ready to see it.

ASK TO SEE YOUR DIVINE TIMING

Are you looking for your divine purpose? Connect to the Creator of All That Is and ask if you're ready to know your divine timing.

Virtues required: Bravery, conviction, courage, determination, faith, hope, and humility.

1. Go up to the Seventh Plane (*see pages 13 and 14*) and make the command (or request), *'Creator of All That Is, if I am ready, show me my divine timing. It is done, it is done, it is done. And so it is.'*

2. Observe your divine timing.

3. When you've finished, rinse yourself off with Seventh-Plane energy and stay connected to it.

If you aren't ready to see your divine timing, you aren't going to get it. You'll go up out of your space to look and get *nothing*. That may be because you have more beliefs to work on and also because your divine timing might be a little overwhelming for you right now.

If you receive information such as: 'You're the only one who can bring a great secret to the world,' then your ego is most likely interfering with your divine connection. But if you see great things beyond yourself, you are without negative ego.

You may also have programs that are blocking you from knowing your divine timing. Energy test for:

'This is my last lifetime.'

'I was made to come here.'

'I hate the Earth.'

Divine Timing Downloads

If you're afraid of seeing your divine timing, maybe there's a reason for it. Maybe you're supposed to do more than you ever imagined. Whatever the case, it's important for you to pull and change your fear of *seeing the future and finding and knowing your divine timing.*

Download:

'I know how to live without the fear of seeing my diving timing.'

'I know how to embrace my divine timing.'

'I know the difference between my divine timing and my ego.'

'I would like memories from my past lives in the highest and best way.'

'I can remember and feel the joy that I brought to this Earth.'

'I can remember the possibilities that were offered to me before I came to this Earth.'

'I know what divine timing is on all levels.'

'I know how to plan for the future.'

'I know what an opportunity is.'

'I know how to take advantage of an opportunity.'

'I know what it feels like to follow through.'

'I know what it feels like to plan for the future.'

'I know how to see the future.'

'I know the divine timing of the Earth.'

'I know that my divine timing is why I am here.'

'I know how to accomplish my divine timing.'

Divine Timing and Free Will

When I tell my students about divine timing, some of them believe it means their life is already planned out and they have to walk that path no matter what. They say, 'If everything's predestined, why am I even here?'

First of all, predestination that was agreed upon before we came here isn't necessarily a bad thing. We agreed to it because we had a reason for coming here and it would help us accomplish what we'd set out to do. It's true that in this life we've the freedom to make our own choices. As tiny sparks of God, we have free agency. And in egotism and stubbornness there are times when we go against the sacred flow of life and, in doing so, wonder why things don't 'go our way.'

But our free will applies to more than just this life. Before we were living this life, we made some decisions about what we would do when we came back to this planet. This is our divine timing. It's something we *want* to do on a soul level, not something we *have* to do.

If you live your life knowing that there's a divine purpose to it all and that you've agreed to play your part, it makes it easier to live on this plane of existence.

The Mission of the Children of the Masters

I've found that there are two kinds of divine timing, depending on the soul essence of a person.

The first is the divine timing of the children of the masters who have been sent here from the Fifth Plane. This sort of divine timing involves acquiring virtues. These children are here to learn the perfect kindness of perfect love.

A child of the masters usually acquires several virtues in a lifetime and carries them to the next in a constant spiral of learning from life to life until the soul ascends to the Fifth Plane and escapes the third dimension. Acquiring these virtues can be the divine timing for each life.

Many of these children talk about how they cannot die until they have accomplished their life mission. This inner desire is so intense that the soul won't quit until the mission is complete. Even death won't stop the divine timing of the soul. If it isn't accomplished in this lifetime, it will be carried over to the next lifetime or to the spirit world of the Fourth Plane.

The Mission of the Ascended Masters

The divine timing of the ascended masters who have come to the Third Plane on a mission is a little more complicated. An awakened master usually has a big list of things to complete – maybe as many as eight divine timings.

An ascended master will feel compelled to heal people and make positive changes to the planet. Their divine timing might be to wake up 1,000,000 souls or to inspire one person who will change the planet. (This motivation isn't normal for a child of the masters until they've been awakened.)

Many masters' divine timing is the Fifth-Plane concept 'Healer, heal thyself.' If so, a healer can assist them, but in the end their divine timing is to heal themselves. Some of my students, for example, have been working on the same illnesses for years. Some of them have had problems since birth. They are doing better, but they aren't completely healed. But that doesn't mean that it won't happen.

There have been many theories as to why a soul would choose to inhabit a body that had physical challenges from birth. Some say that it's because of karma. Some say that the soul chooses the body as a spiritual lesson or to teach the parents unconditional love. But I believe that there's another reason: I believe that some people have created their own sicknesses just so they can heal them.

Unresolved Energy

Because ascended masters have been here many times before, they have the opportunity to meet souls they've known in another time and place. These might be from soul families that are also from the Fifth Plane or might be from past lives.

If these masters have any unresolved energy with any of these souls, they'll have the opportunity to clear it when they meet. The unfinished business may stem from a past-life relationship. Whatever it is, the pair will have the opportunity to meet again in the next life and repair the karma between them. In many instances, people get into relationships to correct karma, and when it's cleared, they outgrow the relationship and move on.

We often meet compatible soul mates based on the energy that we remember from other times and places, and this explains why some of us have more than one soul mate in a lifetime. For example, I've been married four times and divorced three times. (Yes, I have a husband for every direction!) Part of the reason I married three of these people was because on a higher level there was unresolved energy with them from another time and place. This doesn't necessarily mean that there was unfinished business on my part; it was also on the part of the other person.

There's another factor that comes into play too: some of us have made agreements to do something special in this life. It is our life's mission. Anyone who gets in the way of this mission will be moved out of the way, and this includes mates who don't share our vision. Helping the planet and doing healings were so important to me that I divorced two of my husbands so I could stay on my path to divine timing. I knew that it couldn't be accomplished unless I did this. In my last divorce I gave up everything I owned except for my business, one rock, one coffee table, and one sauna. I knew that everything could be replaced, because I'd found something that made me happy. Watching people wake up and learn to do healings made me very happy.

The reason I'm divorced from all three of these men is that the unresolved issues between us were resolved. Each one of them taught me things about myself and helped me to a higher consciousness. Difficult as some of those relationships were, in their own way each helped me to awaken as a spiritual person.

My current relationship is with my divine life partner. I say this because he shares my vision and has the same divine timing as I do. A divine life partner is different than a compatible soul mate. This is someone who has mastered this existence before and has the same divine timing as their mate.

When two souls have been together on the Fifth Plane, they'll look for one another when they go into a human incarnation in order to complete their divine timing here on Earth. There's one particular energy signature that they're searching for. They seem to know what that person looks like and if they share the same path it's almost inevitable that they will meet.

I know that I'm with my assigned divine-timing partner. I believe that when Guy and I met, the heavens opened up and we remembered one another and fell in love all over again.

Having said this, it's important to know that not everyone needs a divine life partner or a compatible soul mate to finish their divine timing. But many of us have the feeling that we don't want to be alone. Do you know why? We weren't meant to accomplish our mission alone. We were meant to accomplish it with the help and support of a special person. This means that part of that mission is to learn how to give our love to one person completely.

Most people of a spiritual nature aren't looking for a soul mate but for the person they're supposed to be with to carry out their mission. Finding this person can be a tricky business.

I know that in order for ThetaHealing to become what it is, I had to have Guy by my side. For so many years before I met him I saw him so clearly and distinctly that I believe he is part of my divine timing.

Collective Divine Timing

Divine timing doesn't just involve the learning process of a single person's soul, it also involves the collective learning process of every soul on the planet. This is why it's important that everyone's personal timing is respected not only for their own sake, but for everyone's sake.

I believe that as we awaken and develop, we come together with our soul family as part of our collective divine timing. Part of our divine truth is coming together as a soul family and working on our belief systems. Belief work helps us to know our divine timing.

On a macrocosmic scale, the Earth itself has its own divine timing. This is why it's a good idea to command that you know what the divine timing of the Earth is on a grand scale. Once you have an awareness of this grand dimension of divinity, it will open up a new understanding that you can use for readings, healings, and manifestations. When you are in a reading or healing, you can ask to see part of the person's divine timing. And when you understand the grand scheme of things, you'll know when to manifest, what to manifest, and how to manifest.

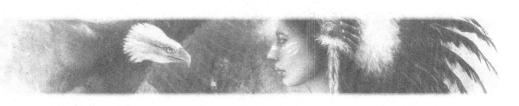

5

THE FOURTH PLANE OF EXISTENCE

The Fourth Plane of Existence is the realm of the spirit. When we die and pass on, our carbon-based body is laid to rest, but our spirit goes forward to the Fourth Plane. If we haven't acquired enough virtues to influence Laws and travel inter-dimensionally, we remain there to learn and evolve, unless we choose to incarnate again on the Third Plane. How many times we go back to the Fourth Plane is entirely up to us and our ability to change and grow.

The Fourth Plane has a totally different time and energy than the Third Plane. What seems like an hour to us is only seconds there.

Fourth-Plane energies have a much higher vibratory rate than those of the Third Plane. In fact, they move faster than the human eye can perceive. Once spirits adjust to the Fourth Plane, they find it much easier to bend the essence of light and vibration.

All the senses are heightened on the Fourth Plane and the spirits there still use some form of nourishment. Male and female essences still exist on the Fourth (and Fifth) Planes and spirits continue to have relationships there.

Spirits on the Fourth Plane reach new heights of learning. The plane itself is divided into sections that teach them about the energies of the First, Second, and Third Planes. It also allows them to influence people on the Third Plane. Many highly evolved guides come from this plane. By helping people on the Third Plane, spirits on the Fourth Plane are able to grow. As they grow, they can obtain the energy that they need to move forward.

DEATH – ONLY THE BEGINNING

When we arrive on the Fourth Plane, we're suddenly able to see thousands of colors. Perception is heightened and every sense accentuated. Everything speeds up. Death is not the end, merely a change in the soul's vibration.

When we step out of this third-dimensional energy, there is no time. Here on Earth time is a blessing, because it tells us when it's time to go home. Getting old is a blessing, but we don't realize this because of the fear of getting older and dying.

A strange thing happens to some people when they get older: they begin to feel a sense of their mortality and turn back to religion. Often this will be the religion they were raised in and, I might add, rejected for the majority of their lives.

The reason for this is that many people fear judgment. Everyone knows that when you die, you are accountable for your life. But it isn't some father-like God sitting on a throne who judges you; the most critical person who looks at your life is *you*. And you'll be much harder on yourself than God would ever be!

The perfect love that creates the universe knows all about you. It knows how you were treated when you were a child. It knows how you felt in every part of your life and it has absolute compassion and loves you without judgment.

WAYWARDS

Some people die feeling that they haven't done well enough in their life. And some spirits with these feelings are afraid to go to the light of creation. They're afraid of being judged. They might have actually done something bad or they might have died a tragic death and feel as though their life is unfinished. Other spirits don't go to God's light because they're trapped by their belief systems. All these spirits are temporarily caught between the Third and the Fourth Planes and are known as 'wayward spirits' or 'waywards.'

Usually a wayward has a problem to solve or some other form of unfinished business. If they can finish this business, they'll instantly go to God's light. Let's say a man commits suicide and becomes a wayward spirit. The reason is that he wants to tell his parents he loves them and he's sorry for what he's done. Until he gets that message through, he'll stay between worlds. Once he is sent to the light, or can overcome his fear and move on, he'll be able to show his love to his parents in a much better way as a guardian angel or guide from the Fourth Plane.

Waywards are in a realm that has no time. A spirit can have died in 1814 and appear in the present without consciously knowing how much time has passed. But eventually every soul finds their way to the Creator. No spirit is ever forgotten. And once the light of the Creator has healed their broken soul, they will pass into the Fourth Plane of Existence.

Some healers are predisposed to send spirits to God's light. They use their own spiritual portal to do so. Sending a spirit to God's light is helping it to go to the Fourth Plane where it can learn and grow. Waywards are almost always young spirits who are still learning and growing.

Usually when a spirit is sent to God's light by a healer, more than one goes through the portal at once. Sometimes thousands of them are sent to the light.

Some healers address a wayward's unfinished business, but others ignore it, because they know that waywards can solve their problems in a better way after they've gone to God's light.

Possession

Because their souls are broken, the inner light of waywards is less than it should be and so they are attracted to the light of living people. When they attach themselves to people, they can drain their energy and make them irritable. Sometimes they undertake various forms of activity so that the people become afraid. Then they can feed on the energy of their fear.

Some people take the energy of a spirit into themselves more than others and this can make them act very strangely. This situation can involve the possession or partial possession of the individual. This is another good reason to send waywards to God's light.

However, I find that in some instances healers confuse viruses, bacteria, and parasites with waywards and alien implants. So they think a person is possessed when actually it's a pathogen that's in the body. They say, 'I was working with a client and I saw that they were possessed. I sent it to the light, but they still have it.'

What they're probably dealing with is a virus that's smart enough to change its energy. A virus hijacks the DNA of a cell and actually possesses the cell. Both viruses and waywards invade the body, but they are very different in the way that they affect a person. Still the healer says, 'Everybody I work on is possessed. There are negative spirits everywhere!'

This may actually mean that there are viral infections that are being passed from person to person. I find that many people have the Epstein-Barr virus and healers can mistake it for other things. I also think that many people confuse parasites and waywards. The person who has the parasite gets the message, 'I am being eaten,' and the healer thinks this means they're being attacked by a spiritual entity.

Since ancient times, people have suspected that diseases stem from unseen organisms or other forces. Even after microbes were visible with a microscope, it took hundreds of years before people accepted that these tiny creatures could cause disease. The germ theory of disease was controversial when it was first developed, although it is the foundation of many aspects of modern medicine.

Even in the 1800s, science didn't believe that viruses or bacteria caused disease or that they were transferred by physical contact. It took someone who intuitively took that leap of faith to say that micro-organisms were passed through contact by the filthy hands of the doctor! This act of bravery came from Ignaz Philipp Semmelweis, who was the first doctor to suggest that doctors should wash their hands with chlorinated lime solutions before working with patients. He could offer no scientific proof of his theory, so it was rejected out of hand. It was not until after his death that his idea was widely accepted and became common practice for doctors. Where did this person get the idea that micro-organisms were passed on in this way? Where did he get the notion that something that he could not see, taste, touch or smell was being passed through physical contact? That's right, it came from his intuition! Just as the intuitive is ridiculed today, so this doctor was ridiculed for his intuition in the past.

All of this illustrates why it's important to ask questions when we're in someone's space in a healing or reading.

If there are many waywards invading a house or area on a continual basis, check to see if there is a portal there, and if so, move it to somewhere harmless (*see page 73*).

If it's a vortex (*see page 69*) that's causing the problem, charge it with positive energy.

THE FALLEN

Long ago, a group of spirits decided that their children on the Third Plane were going home: they would force them to transcend to the Fifth Plane. Of course when they attempted this, they broke the Law of Free Agency and their ability to create was gone, although they retained some lesser powers. Despite this, to this day they think that if they can get enough spirits together, they can break the Law of Free Agency, and they are on this planet right now recruiting spirits to their way of thinking. They are known as 'the fallen.'

Our ancestors called these spirits 'demons.' They can step onto the Third Plane and cause trouble on it, but have a difficult time getting back out of it once they get in. They are powerful beings, but nothing is more powerful than the Creator. An awakened master can command the fallen to leave and there will be no argument if their sacred names are used against them.

However, when some people send these beings to God's light, they do it in a submissive way, and this doesn't work well. The command should be: '*Creator! Send this spirit to the light!*' and it should be said with authority, power, and conviction.

One of my students came into contact with one of the fallen in one of my classes. I could tell she was having a very difficult time meditating and when I asked her what she was doing, she told me she'd been sending love to an evil spirit for over an hour so that it would go to the light, but it wasn't working! She was very frustrated. I told her that the spirit was rejecting her overtures of love and that she had to send it to the light with authority. Then I commanded to know the spirit's sacred name. Using that name, I commanded that it be sent to God's light, visualized it being sucked up by my spiritual portal and made sure that it went all the way to the light.

The fallen and some wayward spirits will attempt to fight you when you are sending them to the light. They want to draw you into conflict, so it's best to avoid that – actually, it's best to avoid talking to them altogether. They can also project weird shapes and say foul things in order to make you fearful. That's why you must be strong, clear, and firm when you witness them being sucked up by a portal and sent on an expressway to the light of creation.

SENDING THE FALLEN TO GOD'S LIGHT

1. Go up to the Seventh Plane (*see pages 13 and 14*) and make the command (not request) with conviction and authority: *'Creator of All That Is, it is commanded that I know this being's sacred name.'*

2. Wait for the vibration of the fallen's sacred name to come to you and then use that vibration to make a second command: *'Creator of All That Is, I command that [give their sacred name] be sent to God's light. Thank you. It is done, it is done, it is done.'*

3. Do not argue with the fallen. They must go to God's light as you have commanded, because you are a spark of God.

4. Witness the fallen being sucked into your spiritual portal and taken all the way to God's light. Continue watching until they become that light.

5. When you choose to break contact, rinse yourself off in Seventh-Plane energy and stay connected to it.

BRIDGING THE PLANES

The Theta brainwave forms a bridge between the planes of existence. When we're in a Theta state, we're much more aware of spiritual energies. This is particularly true when we're asleep and dreaming. I've communicated with all kinds of spiritual energies in this way, but I'd never physically touched one of them until one night in New Delhi, India.

At the end of a long day of teaching I went to sleep and dreamed that a beautiful Indian woman was floating above me. Only the top half of her was visible; the rest just kind of faded out. In my dream, I reached up and grabbed the bottom part of her misty spirit essence and held on. Why I did this I don't know, but as soon as I did, I was fully awake.

Now there have been times when I've awakened to find spirits floating above me, but this time I found that my hands were clenched around the spirit and I was holding on to her for dear life. She was flapping around like a kite in the wind, fighting to get loose from my grip and becoming more and more panicky.

I woke Guy and told him, 'Quick, turn on the light!'

As light filled the room, I saw I was holding on to the lower torso of a beautiful Indian girl. The rest of her was trailing off like Casper the ghost. It was as if I'd bridged the planes and pulled her out of my dream from the Fourth Plane to the Third Plane. She was still struggling, desperate to get away. I let go of her and she took off and flashed out of the room.

I'd caught a ghost with my hands. What an amazing experience!

SPIRITUAL DNA

The Fourth Plane provides access to our ancestors in spirit. Some intuitive healers learn to create an opening to heal people with these ancestor spirits. Healers who are called shamans and medicine men often use spirits and ancestors to aid them in healing. As well as using their ancestors' wisdom, they give the client herbs suggested by ancestral tradition. In this way they form an equation between the Second, Third, and Fourth Planes of Existence. Once a child of the masters understands the Fourth Plane of Existence, they will reach the level of the shaman. Healers who understand the specific healing energy from the Fourth Plane are, however, restricted by the obligations of consciousness that are an inherent part of it.

When children of the masters go to the Fourth Plane between lifetimes, they learn not only from their ancestors there but also from their DNA descendants who are living on the Third Plane. This means that one of our ancestors from the Fourth Plane can in fact look at our life at any time to see what we're learning from our experience here. Knowing that your life can be looked at makes you view your existence here a little differently. When God told me that my life was going to be an open book and people would use it as a reference, I knew that I should live it accordingly.

What isn't working for you in your life? Often it's your DNA that's against you and you may not know it. This is why it's important to uncover the ancestral legacy that's come down to you in your DNA.

Our Ancestors and Their Legacy

Our DNA holds the memories of every ancestor in our genetic line. These records have incredible knowledge in them and can leave a discernible legacy. For instance, when a genetic ancestor leaves many negative beliefs in the DNA, they usually center on one person in the family. This person often has a messy house or is the heaviest in the family because of all the beliefs they're carrying. The toxic thoughts in the body accumulate as fat cells.

Scientists have claimed that 80 percent of the DNA inside us is 'junk.' But I feel that within this 80 percent of unknown DNA there's vast knowledge which, once understood, will give us the ability to do amazing things.

We all came here with a DNA code, and this code doesn't tell us *what* we are as much as *who* we are. Who we are is the result of every experience that our ancestors had before us, and this knowledge is obtainable.

Who were your ancestors? Obviously they were survivors and they knew how to keep going no matter what. They had the program that no matter what happened in life they could survive it. This is why you have a real need to survive within your DNA. Some ancestors were leaders and some were followers, so you have these selections to choose from. Some found that loving someone hurt too much, so they learned not to love anyone. Others learned that the only thing that got them through was love.

I believe that a lot of our personality now is dependent on what our ancestors did before us. For instance, I didn't grow up with my father, but I still inherited some genetic patterns from him. At first, I didn't like this idea at all, because my father has some attributes that I don't care for. Naturally, I didn't want to pick up any of the negative things from him, but as I reflected on my ancestral line I could see that there were a lot of good things there as well.

I know that I came into this world with kindness on a genetic level. My father is very kind, but my mother had genetic material of a different sort. I believe that the strongest genetic belief will win out, and in this case, the kindness was passed down to me.

My father taught me to work hard and this tendency had been passed down to him from past generations. He came from good, strong, frontier people. My great-great grandmother was a midwife who delivered babies in Utah.

All my life, I've had the habit of sleeping with my feet out of the bedcovers and so does my father. I never knew this until recently.

Whenever I can, I like to go barefoot, and I've found out that I have lines of grandmothers who liked to go barefoot too.

I didn't realize how much Native American blood I had until I took my DNA admixture blood test for ratios of European, Asian, sub-Saharan African, and Native American. I found that I was part Native American and the rest European, just as my mother had said.

I've realized that I think a lot like a Native American. Even though I'm only part Native American, I still raised my family like a tribe. To this day, we help each other with everything. When my granddaughter Jenaleighia was born, the whole family took care of her. We all want our family members to be close and stay in the tribe.

Before I met Guy, I moved 39 times. Since then I've moved three times in 17 years, but I've circled the globe many times on an almost constant travel schedule. I might complain about traveling, but when I get to where I'm going, I put a flower in a vase, hang my hat, and that is home. Where did this 'moving energy' come from? It's in my DNA! I can move into different environments very well, just as my European pioneering folk and Native American ancestors did.

Many feelings have been locked into this Earth from the strong emotions of generation upon generation of humans who came before us. Through belief work, we can release these feelings, even from our genetic line.

This is why we do belief work: to free our ancestors from the negative emotions that they experienced when they were alive, so that they can be free of them in the spirit world of the Fourth Plane through our DNA connection.

Belief Work with the Ancestors

As we interact with Fourth-Plane energies, we are interacting with our future DNA, which is represented by our children, and the DNA of the past, which is represented by our ancestors. As we change our DNA programs, this helps both ancestors and children to progress to the next level of their development.

When we progress spiritually, this energetic influence goes into the huge DNA of our family line and is passed backward into the past and forward into the future. This means that if we learn something important, our ancestors of the Fourth Plane learn it as well.

When we do belief work, we are replacing the beliefs of several generations of ancestors at least. If we were to ask the Creator how far a belief went back, the reply might be, 'Twelve generations.'

We know that the morphogenetic field is an energy signature of knowledge that flows through the DNA and tells it what to do. It tells a baby's cells how many legs, how many feet, and how many hands it's going to have. The morphogenetic field also holds genetic ancestral memories that go back at least seven generations. When we want to create a change in our ancestral memory, we should command this change for seven generations back and seven generations forward from the womb.

CREATING A CHANGE IN OUR ANCESTRAL ENERGY

Virtues required: Compassion and kindness.

1. Go up to the Seventh Plane (*see pages 13 and 14*) and make the command: *'Creator of All That Is, it is commanded [or requested] that love be sent to this person as a baby in the womb seven generations forward and seven generations back. Thank you. It is done, it is done, it is done.'*

2. Go up and witness the Creator's unconditional love surrounding the baby, whether it is you, your own child, or your parents.

3. Witness love filling the womb and watch as it envelopes the fetus and eliminates all poisons, toxins, and negative emotions for seven generations forward and seven generations back.

4. Surround the person with love through their whole life and beyond.

5. Rinse yourself off with Seventh-Plane energy and stay connected to it.

The Genetic Level and the Ancestors

The genetic level of belief work has a direct connection with the Fourth Plane. It consists of the genetic code of our ancestors and the genetic programs of the DNA. These exist on the Fourth Plane as an actual intelligence in a marriage with the Law of DNA.

Within the DNA record, there are:

• genetic beliefs that are active in our life. These can have positive or negative effects.

• genetic beliefs that are dormant. If these were activated, they could work to our benefit or detriment.

When we are healing, we affect the healing 94 to 96 percent with our own belief system. The person being healed only has to believe 4 to 6 percent that it is possible.

When you do enough belief work with a person, you open up the possibility that they will heal. A belief-work session may open the possibility of a healing for only 10 minutes, but the person may heal in those 10 minutes.

When you witness a healing, it is best to go up and talk to God to see how the person's body has responded to it.

Ask the Creator, 'Did they take the healing?'

God says, 'Yes.'

Then you ask, 'How much?'

God says, 'Just a little bit.'

So you do more belief work and then do another healing.

Then you ask God, 'How much did they take the healing?'

God says, 'They took the healing 50 percent.'

This means that it is possible that they are completely healed.

If we can create the possibility that healing can happen, we can make changes. With the guidance of the Creator, we can go back and change the past. If I was going to work on diabetes, for example, and it was caused by a genetic predisposition, I would still work on all the person's beliefs about diabetes, but the key would be to go back to the original ancestor where the diabetes started and change the past. If someone had cancer, for instance, we could change their genetic predisposition for cancer by going back to where it started, perhaps four generations ago, and changing the beginning of the anomaly in the DNA of their ancestor.

REPAIRING A GENETIC DEFECT

With knowledge of the genetic record, you can find a genetic defect and follow it back to the time when it was created by one of your ancestors. Then God can change it by using the DNA of one of the other genetic lines. Once the defect has been changed, this energy is brought forward to the present. This has worked on many babies in Theta.

1. Go up to the Seventh Plane (see pages 13 and 14) and make the command: 'Creator of All That Is, take me back in time to when this genetic defect was created. Thank you. It is done, it is done, it is done.'

2. Witness going back in time to when the genetic defect was created.

3. Witness the defect being changed using another genetic line and brought forward in time to the present.

4. Witness the changes being integrated into the body in the present through every cell in the body, making the body strong.

5. Once the process is finished, rinse yourself off in Seventh-Plane energy and stay connected to it.

Retrieving Ancestral Information

We can clear, shift, and change the genetic beliefs that are obvious to us, but what about those that are unknown to us? And what of genetic attributes that we'd like to awaken and embrace?

What if we could go back to an ancestor's life and bring their positive attributes forward into our own life? After all, this information is already sleeping in our DNA. What if we could go back and understand our ancestors in a deeper way and bring back skills that took them years to learn? These too are dormant in our DNA – we just need to reawaken them. We can bring these energies forward into the present so that we have our ancestors' attributes without having to create them ourselves.

You have already inherited attributes that have become evident, but what if you could go back and understand your ancestors in a deeper way and bring back to this time things that took them years to learn? This is an instinctual ability that is dormant in our DNA, which permits us to reach backward into the past and bring forward positive attributes from our ancestors.

What is important is that we are aware of ancestral beliefs and attributes that are beneficial and unbeneficial. Then we can awaken those that are positive and change those that are negative.

Going back and retrieving attributes from your ancestors can save you a lot of time and trouble. I've retrieved bravery, because I felt I lacked it. Some people think I'm very brave, but what I have is courage. I can face fear and go forward, but I wanted to be able to have no fear – I wanted bravery. So God took me back and I retrieved it from my ancestors. Now I'm integrating it into my life. I'm doing things without feeling and overcoming fear. I've made up my mind to do it and I'm going to do it.

I trust the answers I get from God and I also trust my intuition. But I still energy test myself, because energy testing can override your own ego to tell you what's really going on in your subconscious mind. Your ego can be your friend or your enemy. You need to keep it in check at all times or you won't be able to work on yourself. There are healers who say they are perfect and that they don't need to do any more work on themselves. As for me, when I'm perfect, I will know when it happens. It's kind of an oxymoron, because we are already perfect – we have the perfect disease, the perfect sickness, in the perfect form. But I always think that we can keep working on ourselves to become a better person.

Everyone has an ego, and this includes our ancestors. I believe it is possible to connect with our ancestors through meditation and create positive results in the process, but we have to be careful. When we go back to an ancestor's life and bring good attributes forward, we don't want to bring back their negative ego as well.

We may also go traveling all around the world to bring back the memories of different times and places. If we feel that a genetic memory is coming back, we need to go up and command that the good information stays and that we can filter out the negative energies.

In order to bring back positive attributes from our ancestors, we can use a crystal layout technique to retrieve the good attributes that are lying dormant in our DNA and magnify them in our life.

The Crystal Layout

A crystal layout is a form of guided meditation using crystals arranged around the body. It is a good example of a marriage of First-Plane crystals with the Fourth-Plane energies of ancestral DNA. It was originally designed for past-life regression, but it wasn't long before we started having people going back to a past life and getting stuck in other times and places as they were coming back. So we learned to take them to the end of a lifetime and resolve all the issues from it by starting the meditation from the Seventh Plane and ending the meditation at the Seventh Plane. This was so successful that we began to use crystal layouts for many different purposes.

Students of ThetaHealing learn how to find the negative things their ancestors passed down to them when they take the 'World Relations' class, using belief work. But the crystal layout here is different in that we are looking for the *good* things that our ancestors have given us.

Take a minute and write down on a piece of paper the good traits that you have in your life right now. What would you like more of? What would you like to magnify? Would you like to be kinder or more considerate?

When people do past-life regression or crystal layouts for past-life information, it doesn't necessarily mean that the experience is going to be about their own past lives. In many instances what they get is a genetic-ancestor experience. We are part of Atanaha, the 'All That Is,' so if we really want to know and experience the memories of everyone who has ever lived, I believe it is possible to do so. But these incarnations are not only human Third-Plane experiences, they can be much more. For instance, you may have been an angel in another incarnation and assisted people in that form, which is a Fifth-Plane experience.

What attributes would you like to retrieve from your ancestors? If you want empathy and unconditional love, you should go to an ancestor who experienced these in their life. You can go back as far as 2,000 years or more, even to the time of Christ. You might find that you are carrying some bizarre things in your DNA memory. Some people find that their ancestors were amazing people and great prophets.

A CRYSTAL LAYOUT FOR RETRIEVING ANCESTRAL INFORMATION

In this kind of crystal layout meditation we use a quartz crystal that is cut in the special shape of a Star of David. However, a piece of clear quartz or opal works as well.

There should always be two people for this exercise: one is the practitioner and one is the client. Avoid doing it alone. Having another person there will make you feel safer and you will need a guide to make sure you move forward with the meditation and retrieve the right information.

When you use crystals in a layout to retrieve information, you should always clear any past-life memories that may be in them. This is because there may be confusion between the memories in the stone and the memories you want to see. Because the molecules in the stones move at a slower rate, this only works for about an hour at a time and then the memories come back into them. Go to the Seventh Plane (*see pages 13 and 14*) and ask to clear the stones of any memories they hold.

Use your proper spiritual name when you go back to do ancestral work. This will help you access archives that hold the memories of everyone that you have been related to.

When you retrieve ancestral virtues, it may feel as though it is your own life that you are experiencing.

1. The client lies down with their head in the south, because this connects them with a strong psychic energy.

2. The practitioner sits behind the client's head, above their crown, and, if the client is comfortable with being touched, gently places both hands on their head. Through this touch, the client is now sharing genetic information with the practitioner. Never touch a client unless they are comfortable with it, but if you understand the workings of this exercise, your touch will train their DNA in how to do the meditation.

3. The quartz crystal in the shape of a Star of David (or the piece of quartz crystal or opal) is placed on the client's third eye, in the middle of their forehead, and the two spherical crystals, called drivers, are held in each hand. If the client wants to get a better view of what is going on in the meditation, they simply move the drivers round in their hands as a way of helping themself focus.

4. The practitioner downloads the quartz crystal and the drivers with the ability to guide the client in the meditation, keep them in a Theta wave, and retain everything that happens in the experience. The crystals therefore act as recorders and every time the client holds them, they will remember the experience in detail.

5. The practitioner leads the client into the meditation.

To give you an idea of what may come up in a meditation like this, here is an example.

Attributes from an Ancestor

Vianna (leads the client into the meditation as follows): Take a deep breath in and imagine the energy coming up through the bottom of your feet. Move up to the top of your head and become a beautiful ball of light. What color is it? [I ask what color the person is envisioning so that I can match their energy.]

Woman: *It is a pink color.*

Vianna: Imagine going up past layers of light, through a golden light, through a thick jelly-like substance and into a tingly white light.

Make the command: '*Creator of All That Is, it is commanded – or requested – that I see and witness this ancestor's life and witness the attributes that are beneficial to me being brought forward into my life. It is done, it is done, it is done.*'

Now imagine going down into the middle of space and time and seeing a doorway. In just a moment we're going to step back into an ancestor's life and you're going to see the things you requested. Are you ready?

One, two, three, step through the door. Look down at your feet. Are you a man or are you a woman?

Woman: *I am a man.*

Vianna: Can you get a sense of what year it is?

Woman: *I am getting the year 1790.*

Vianna: Tell me what was the first significant event of this person's life.

Woman: *They came across the sea.*

Vianna: Where were they coming to?

Woman: *Scotland.*

Vianna: Okay, move forward in time in this life. Did they make it okay across the sea?

Woman: *They did.*

Vianna: So does this man have a family?

Woman: *Yes.*

Vianna: And children?

Woman: *Yes.*

Vianna: And he loves them?

Woman: *Yes, but he came across the waters first.*

Vianna: So did they catch up with him? Did his family come later?

Woman: *Yes.*

Vianna: So, you're looking for the energy that he has with regard to his family – the empathy, the unconditional love, and the sense of working well with people. Does he have these things?

Woman: *Yes.*

Vianna: Do people like him?

Woman: *Yes.*

Vianna: Is he strong?

Woman: *Yes, he's very strong.*

Vianna: Has he a religion of any kind?

Woman: *Yes. He is a Protestant.*

Vianna: Okay, I want you to move forward in his life to the next significant event.

Woman: *He's holding a baby.*

Vianna: Is there anything else you want to tell me?

Woman: *No, no, it doesn't seem to be important.*

Vianna: Okay, I want you to move to the next significant event.

Woman: *Ah, the baby grows up. I have become her.*

Vianna: Does she have the same attributes as her father?

Woman: *Yes, she does. Yes.*

Vianna: Okay, I want you to go to the completion of his life and the completion of her life.

Woman: *She moves to Australia.*

Vianna: Okay, so I want you to imagine watching her life right through to the end and resolving all of the issues, and tell me when you're done. How does she die?

Woman: *She dies of old age, but she's still quite young. It's because she has struggled a lot.*

Vianna: So she dies from natural causes?

Woman: *Yes.*

Vianna: Can you see her struggles?

Woman: *Yes. It was harsh – it was a harsh land.*

Vianna: Now I want you to imagine her going up between lives as she resolves her issues. Does she go into God's light?

Woman: *Well, she stays around for a while because she's worried about her children and grandchildren.*

Vianna: So how long does it take her to go to God's light?

Woman: *She stays for 30 years and then she leaves.*

Vianna: Okay. Now do I have permission to make sure that you bring forward all of her genetic lessons of kindness, and empathy, and unconditional love, and the energy of working well with other people? Do I have permission to bring them up through your DNA and magnify them 10 times?

Woman: *Yes.*

Vianna: Take a deep breath in. Good girl. I want you to command that *'these attributes, abilities, and virtues be brought forward into my DNA, through every ancestor into me now, magnified 10 times, that my body fully accepts them and they are allowed to come forward. Creator, teach my body that it deserves them. Witness these energies being brought through all the lines of my people to me.'* Tell me when it is done.

Woman: *It is done.*

Vianna: Okay, I want you to imagine stepping out through the door. Go into the universe and go back to that tingly white light. Feel unconditional love go through every cell of your body. Good. I want you to come back here, to this time, to this date. You are in a ThetaHealing class in Idaho. Take a deep breath in and open your eyes.

Be sure to allow the client to see a few significant events in their ancestor's life and to follow them through that life all the way to their death. Make sure the ancestor goes to the light. Let them resolve any issues between lives. You may also move on to look at the life of one of their children because of the DNA connection.

Then make sure the client brings the attributes they need all the way through the DNA into the present day. Take them back through the door, then back to the Creator. Make sure they arrive back safely and soundly. They will likely remember the experiences and energy of their ancestor's life all day long. This energy will go down to their children too.

Can you bring back attributes from a person if you're not related to them? No, but you can feel those attributes and download them from the Creator. (When attributes come down through genetics they are felt in a different way.)

Each time you do a crystal layout you should come closer to a point where you no longer need the tools of the crystals and the drivers, but use them at the start because they will keep you in a Theta brainwave and will retain everything that happens in the experience.

Here's another example:

Vianna: What attributes are you after?

Man: *Self-discipline and enthusiasm.*

Vianna: Okay, it is the intention of both the practitioner and the client to retrieve these attributes. Imagine yourself in a ball of light. What color is it?

Man: *It's blue.*

Vianna: Go up to the Seventh Plane of Existence and make the command: '*Show us the life of the ancestor who has these attributes.*'

We're going to walk through a door to go to the life of an ancestor who has these abilities. One, two, three, step through the door and find yourself in this ancestor's life. Look down at your feet. Are you a man or a woman?

Man: *A man.*

Vianna: Where is this and can you see what you're wearing?

Man: *Sandals and sheepskin.*

Vianna: How long ago was this?

Man: *It was 3,000 years ago.*

Vianna: Look at this man's life. Touch, taste, and feel his life experience. Go to the next significant event of his life.

Man: *He's taking part in some kind of ceremony.*

Vianna: What's he like? Is he fun? Is he nice?

Man: *He has lots of humor and is a very strong, macho kind of man.*

Vianna: Is he married?

Man: *Yes, he has two wives and lots of children.*

Vianna: Is he happy?

Man: *Yes. He is a happy person.*

Vianna: I want you to feel his faith. What is his faith like?

Man: *He is a believer.*

Vianna: Can you feel the energy of his faith?

Man: *Yes. It isn't faith but knowing.*

Vianna: I want you to move through his life to the time of his death. How does he die?

Man: *It is something to do with water. I see him lying on a large rock. He has a silent death.*

Vianna: I want you to go up after his death and see that he resolves any issues that were in his life. I want you to imagine him going to the light. I want you to see his children.

Now do I have permission to make sure that you bring forward all of his faith, self-discipline, and enthusiasm? Do I have permission to bring them up through your DNA and magnify them 10 times?

Man: *Yes.*

Vianna: Okay, I want you to command '*that these attributes, abilities, and virtues be brought forward into my DNA, into me now, magnified 10 times, that my body fully accepts them and they are allowed to come forward. Creator, teach my body that it deserves them. Witness these energies being brought through all the lines of my people to me.*' Tell me when it is done.

Man: *It is done.*

Vianna: Walk back through the door, go back to the Creator of All That Is, and open your eyes.

Virtues from an Ancestor

Here's an example of bringing forward virtues:

Vianna: What virtue would you like to bring forward from one of your ancestors?

Man: *I protect the innocent, so I would like to have courage.*

Vianna: You already have courage. Just coming to a metaphysical class takes courage. Just going through American customs takes courage! So would you like to have courage or bravery?

Man: *All right, I would like to have bravery.*

Vianna: Bravery means you can act without fear. Let's go find an ancestor who had this virtue.

Take a deep breath in and imagine the energy coming up through the bottom of your feet. Move up to the top of your head and become a beautiful ball of light. What color is it?

Man: *It is blue.*

Vianna: Imagine going up past layers of light, through a golden light, through a thick jelly-like substance and into a tingly white light. Make the command: '*Creator of All That Is, it is commanded – or requested – that I see and witness the life of an ancestor who had incredible bravery* *in their DNA and the attributes that are beneficial to me being brought forward to my life. Thank you. It is done, it is done, it is done.'*

Now imagine going down into the middle of space and time and seeing a doorway. In just a moment we're going to step back into the life of an ancestor who had bravery. Are you ready?

One, two, three, step through the door. Look down at your feet. Are you a man or a woman? Where are you at in history? Are you many generations back or only a few?

Man: *I am a man. This is many generations back and I am wearing boots.*

Vianna: Listen to the name that people are calling you. Where do you live?

Man: *The man is an amazing fighter!*

Vianna: Is he using a sword?

Man: *A lightweight beautiful sword embossed with gold.*

Vianna: What is he fighting for?

Man: *Freedom. He is fighting for the freedom of his people.*

Vianna: Feel the energy of this person. He has not only bravery but a love of freedom and many other qualities as well. Move forward in his life. Can you see how he dies?

Man: *He dies in battle.*

Vianna: Does he have children? Did he pass on this bravery to one of his children?

Man: *He died for his children.*

Vianna: I want you to see that bravery in his children.

Man: *Yes, I see it.*

Vianna: Make the command that this bravery comes forward through all the generations to you, to be reinforced and magnified in this time and place. Are you ready?

Man: *Yes.*

Vianna: Now I want you to leave this place. See everything in this man's life resolved and go back through the door. Go back to the Creator's energy of light and love.

You said you protected the innocent, correct? Now I want you to go back to that tingly white light and go into your cells and go to a lifetime where you learned to protect the innocent. Tell me where you end up. Where are you?

Man: *I don't understand it – there's only light in this place, only light.*

Vianna, to class: This means that he learned to protect the innocent before he ever came here to Earth, when he was a being of light. [*To man:*] Now imagine that this energy of protecting the innocent is brought forth from this place of light and magnified within you. This light has other qualities too. What other qualities do you feel there are here?

Man: *I'm not sure.*

Vianna: This being of light feels very kind. Is he kind? Are you safe?

Man: *I can't contain the energy of this being!*

Vianna: Would you like the download that you can contain this energy?

Man: *Yes, please.*

Vianna: Okay. Now bring the positive qualities you had when you were this being of light forward into your DNA. Your cells are safe and your body is full of joy. Go back to that tingly white light, take a deep breath in and find yourself back, safe and strong.

As you can see, I told him to go back into his DNA history and he went back to when he was a being of light on the Fifth Plane. I also told him to find where he got the qualities that he already had, and he went back to a time when he was a spiritual energy. He did this by following his DNA backward. So he went back to an ancestor who was a swordsman, then he went back to the spiritual world when he was an angel. Not everyone experiences all of their lives on the Third Plane. Some of us have spent many lives on the Fifth Plane of Existence as beings of light.

SHAMANISM

As mentioned earlier, some intuitive healers use the spirits and ancestors of the Fourth Plane to aid them in healing. They are known as shamans.

Shamanism is one of the oldest professions in the history of humanity. Shamanistic traditions have existed since prehistoric times; at one time, every culture had some form of shamanistic practice. Shamans were the first to experiment with influencing spiritual energy and they practiced precursors of many of the modalities that we use today. Shamanism is also likely to be the forerunner of religion, not to mention religious thought. Over time, modern religions, science, and social practices have replaced many of these ancient traditions.

Shamans are said to transverse the Axis Mundi, the cosmic axis linking heaven and Earth. They give people healing or herbs suggested by the wisdom of the ancestors. In this way they make an equation between the Second, Third, and Fourth Planes.

Shamans are credited with the ability to connect to spirit animals, manipulate the weather, interpret dreams, undertake astral projection and journeying, and travel to the upper and lower worlds to commune with spiritual energies. In its traditional form, shamanism includes soul fragment retrieval and shapeshifting into other forms to speak to spirits and to draw, or 'pull out,' disease into the shaman themselves or into another life-form, such as a tree, or the Earth. Shamanism is a dualistic practice – the practitioner has the choice to use it for good or ill.

Some healers are instinctual shamans in that they attempt to pull other people's difficulties into themselves. This may be from a genetic memory, but it may also be that as the intuition develops there is a natural connection to the energy of shamanism.

Because all of our experiences matter to the soul, it won't release this tendency with belief work. For instance, if a small child is in pain, the soul is likely going to help the child in any way it can. So it's better to download the knowledge of how to send the pain to God's light. Do this with:

'If I take on anyone's sickness, beliefs, or pain, it is
automatically converted and sent to God's light.'

Spirit Guides and Animal Totems

In ancient times, we lived closely with wild animals and venerated each
species. Ancient peoples around the world had belief systems based upon
a pantheon of animals. Egyptian mythology started out this way, as did
the belief systems of some of the tribes in India. Over time, the gods
and goddesses began to take the shape of men and women, though some
cultures viewed their gods as having both human and animal attributes.
The Celtic god Cernunnos and the Indian god Ganesh are good examples.
In Greek mythology, there was a consistent theme of fusion between man
and animal, as expressed in the centaur (half-man, half-horse), and the
Medusa, with her tresses of snake-hair. Animals were even morphed with
other animals, as in the Chimera.

One of the most ancient examples of this fusion with animals comes
from a cave in Lascaux, France. A painting there depicts a figure wearing
the skin of an animal and a headdress of horns. This eerily resembles the
depiction of Cernunnos on an ancient cauldron found in Denmark. The
interesting thing is that the illustrations are more than 20,000 years apart!

In the ancient world, rituals were performed in which men and women
would seek out a 'totem' or spiritual animal guide. This guide was viewed
as a source of strength and enlightenment. The individual would seek
to take upon themselves the attributes of their animal guide in order to
benefit from their wisdom and strength. Shamans used the spiritual energy
from animal totems to intensify their own abilities in all kinds of ways – in
prophecy, healing, wooing a lover, and winning a battle.

Animal totems also included mythological creatures such as dragons
and unicorns and the thunderbird of the Native Americans, all of which
were considered to have magical powers.

The wisdom and power of an animal totem can still be invoked
when needed. The 'power animal' is found through meditation, prayer,
and drumming ceremonies. Then the person takes the essence of the
animal within.

Some Native Americans believe everyone has at least one power animal. Some tribes believe that we have as many as seven to nine.

Many American tribes also believe that all animals have a purpose and teach us through their physical and spiritual presence. In my experience, wild animals will send spiritual messages in physical form. They will do something out of the ordinary to get a message to you.

Shapeshifting

Shamanic practices around the world involve shapeshifting – shamans either changing their body into the form of an animal or sending their consciousness into the body of an animal.

The practice of changing the physical form into an animal is known in the Navaho nation, as well as in Mexican and South American native cultures.

In the other way of shapeshifting, sending the consciousness into the body of an animal, the shaman or medicine person connects to the animal through the collective soul energy of the species. Most animals have an individual soul, but it is possible to connect to the collective spiritual energy and see what it has to teach you. It is also possible to send your consciousness into a wild animal to cohabit with it for a time. The spirit of the animal is not pushed out; rather, it is a shared experience for animal and person.

Are shapeshifters real? Of course they are! Why do I say this? Because I believe that it *is* possible to send our consciousness into animals and see through their eyes. I have sent my consciousness into wolves to look through their eyes as they hunted. I also believe there are people who have the ability to change their features. There are people who can live off other people's energy too, and this may be where the legends of vampires come from.

You can shapeshift spiritually into an animal by using a crystal layout. When you do this, always say, '*I agree to do this in the Creator's way, a good way.*'

SPIRITUAL SHAPESHIFTING

In this exercise, two people work together. One is the practitioner and the other is the client. There should always be two people! Avoid doing this exercise alone. With another person there, you will feel safer and be guided to move forward.

This is a crystal layout using a quartz crystal, which is placed on the third eye, and two spherical crystals, called drivers, which are held in each hand.

1. Use the Seventh-Plane meditation (*see pages 13 and 14*) to clear the stones of any memories that are in them.

2. The practitioner downloads the crystal and the drivers with the ability to guide the client in the meditation, keep them in a Theta wave, and retain everything that happens in the experience with the animal.

3. The client lies down with their head in the south, because this connects them with a strong psychic energy.

4. The practitioner sits behind the client's head, above the crown, and gently places both hands on their head.

5. The practitioner leads the client into the meditation as follows:

'We are going to spiritually shapeshift into an eagle [or an animal of your choice]. Center yourself in your heart, take a deep breath in and imagine energy coming up through the bottom of your feet, into your body, and up through all the chakras. Go out through your crown chakra and project your consciousness out past the stars to the universe.

Imagine going up beyond the universe, past layers of light, through a golden light, past a thick jelly-like substance and into a tingly white light.

Make the command to the Creator of All That Is: 'It is commanded [or requested] that I shapeshift into an eagle. It is done, it is done, it is done.'

Now imagine going down into the middle of space and time and seeing a doorway.

One, two, three, step through the door. Look around you and find the animal.

Take another deep breath in. You are now in the animal's space. What does it feel like? What does it feel like to be the eagle, to soar and see through the eyes of the eagle? Feel its heartbeat, its strength, and its vigor. Experience this for a while. What do you see?

Are you ready to come back?

Now envision stepping back though the door.

Go into the universe and back to that tingly white light of the Seventh Plane. Feel unconditional love go through every cell of your body.

Come back to this time and place. Take a deep breath in and open your eyes.'

This connection with an animal will give you a great sense of its health, strength, and spiritual essence.

The universe is always communicating with you. Your power animal will often show up in your life or in your dreams to guide you.

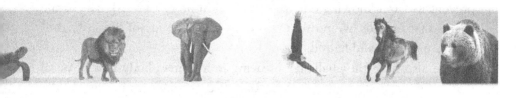

6

THE THIRD PLANE OF EXISTENCE

The Third Plane of Existence is where animals and humans exist in a symphony of life. The elements of the seven planes – minerals, photosynthesis, spiritual energy, and physical energy – all come together on this plane to make us what we are. This is the plane of protein-based molecules, carbon-based structures, and amino acid-based chains. These organic compounds are the basis of life here.

The Third Plane is where we learn to control our body, thoughts, and feelings. This is the plane of dreams, ideas, and decisions. Complex beings of the Third Plane, such as humans and animals, have imagination and great problem-solving abilities. We humans often think that we're more evolved than the beings of the First and the Second Planes and the animals with whom we co-exist on this plane. Perhaps this is because we have a well-developed ego, an instinct that was given to us to help us survive and achieve. Since egotism thrives on the Third Plane, we must control this aspect of ourselves.

It is on this plane in fact that we have the challenge of being governed by emotions, instinctual desires, and passions. How we balance our emotions will dictate how well we are able to access the other planes and move freely through them to create health.

In the creation of our own reality, we have formed the illusions of programs, thought-forms, and collective consciousness that keep our thoughts bound to this plane. This may mean that some of our physical, mental, and spiritual abilities are blocked. Negative belief systems can prevent us from knowing our true abilities. In order to break free of the chains that bind us, we must concentrate upon the joy of life instead of fear, resentment, and hatred.

We also have the challenge of being in a human body in a physical world. Our physical body is a reflection of everything we believe. In the same context, everything that is going on in our life is also going on in our body. The way we look and how we feel are a perceived identity that is created in the illusion of the Third Plane. If we have too many negative beliefs, or positive beliefs creating a negative, it causes an energy fracture in the All That Is of what we are. In order to make us aware of these energy fractures, the Creator has given us illness. In order to transcend illnesses of all kinds, we must change our beliefs.

To manifest change, we must break free from our limited Third-Plane consciousness. It is important to create a cosmic consciousness, an understanding that we are more than a physical body in a physical world. This is one of the reasons why we go up so quickly through the planes of existence in the Seventh-Plane meditation – so that we're not influenced by the negative beliefs that are in the physical body, on the physical Earth, or in the physical universe that we travel through while on a pure Theta wave. In this way we avoid the heavy thoughts that are on this plane and outside the confines of the Earth and the physical body.

We create our life based on our fears, doubts, disbelief, resentment, and anger, as well as the positive feelings and emotions that become virtues. While we are on this planet, the challenge is to outweigh the negative feelings with the positive, not only to have health, happiness, and joy, but also to transcend to the realms of enlightenment.

Because the Third Plane of Existence is the school of Fifth Plane of Existence energies, we are divine in nature and can easily be taught and reminded how to use a Seventh-Plane essence. In order to graduate from the Third Plane of Existence, the human 'student' must learn this. The masters from the Fifth Plane have come here to help their human Third-Plane students/children back to the Fifth Plane of Existence, but they must regain their knowledge of the virtues.

CHILDREN OF THE FIFTH PLANE

We may think that we're physically on the Third Plane, but we actually exist on all of the planes of existence. In reality, as explained earlier, we are children of the Fifth Plane.

We actually seem to have some conscious recollection of this. It explains why many people believe they are 'children of God,' because we have a spiritual father and mother on the Fifth Plane. These spiritual parents give us encouragement, compassion, and advice. They are high masters from the Fifth Plane of Existence.

To meet your spiritual parents, it's best to go through the Creator of All That Is. This is because once you've been purified by the essence of the Seventh Plane, you'll be better able to communicate with them. They will guide you to become a master yourself.

If you often feel as though you don't belong here on Earth, that it is too harsh, that people are cruel, and you feel incredibly homesick and miss your spiritual family, then you may be a Fifth-Plane ascended master. Remember, masters from the Fifth Plane have come here to help their Third-Plane children back to the Fifth Plane. If you know you have incredible abilities and a strong connection to the Creator, you may be a master waking up to help the Earth.

Whether you are an ascended master or a child of the masters, you are learning by acquiring positive virtues.

THE DIVINE HUMAN BODY

All things in existence are divine in nature, and this includes the human body. It is the way that our spirit experiences this plane. The cells in our body are working tirelessly to give us this life experience. Our lungs giggle and celebrate each time we take a breath of air. Our liver and other organs are singing to one another. Do we stop to feel this celebration? We forget we are here to breathe, to laugh, to live in this beautiful body. We should remind ourselves that this is a wonderful plane to exist on. But we are here to learn as a spiritual being and some of us still learn through pain and suffering. This is one of our spiritual challenges on this plane: to learn without creating suffering and to experience joy.

Even though we're all connected to All That Is, we often don't see ourselves in this way. Everything we eat and experience here on Earth is designed to keep us here in the physical body. As our spirit matures in this human body, the Earth becomes our cradle. Our spirit likes being in this cradle and if ever we go several days without angry thoughts and begin to make a spiritual connection, we start thinking, *What's going to happen to me if I become enlightened? Am I going to change? Am I going to evolve? Will I die?* Or, even worse, *Will I be left alone? Will my friends and relatives change with me?* As soon as these worries come in, we rescue ourselves from spiritual enlightenment.

As spiritual beings within the sometimes restrictive confines of the physical body, we are faced with the challenge of overcoming these illusionary restrictions and taking responsibility for our human body and all its systems, including those that are spiritual in nature. This is our challenge: to overcome these perceived illusionary restrictions and flourish with the human body, and thus change our perception of our existence within it.

If we viewed the processes of the human body as sacred, it would mean that we were walking around in a miracle of God's bioengineering. It would mean that there were no mistakes in the universe and all of the body's functions had a divine purpose. It would also mean that there was no separation between what was physical and what was spiritual. Our challenge is to start to think this way.

Spiritual and Physical Integration

As we saw earlier, in order to come into a human body, a multi-dimensional spirit goes through a spiritual portal. When the sperm impregnates the egg inside the womb, there's a flash of light that is conception. At this moment, a spiritual portal is formed that joins the Third Plane to a dimension from the Fourth or Fifth Plane. This portal is composed of pure intelligence (thought), which brings the soul into the newly formed fetus.

If the vibration of the Fifth-Plane spirit that comes into the baby is too high, the fetus may miscarry or the baby become physically weakened. It can also be that the frequency is too high for the body of the mother.

If the baby survives this union of Third- and Fifth-Plane energies, it may be sickly because of the mixture of two very different vibrations. This sometimes happens when an ascended master comes into a human body and it is why intuitive people are sometimes sickly at first. For an ascended master, it can be a challenge to function in a human body without destroying it.

It takes a while for children who have fresh spiritual energies to get used to the human body, but it's still an incredibly magical experience for them. Even as a young child I knew that our physical form was only a small part of us. I knew that I was wearing my skin and that there was more to me than just my body. When I was about seven, our neighbor's baby would escape through their basement window and waddle around naked in the yard. As my mother watched, she would become judgmental toward the parents, saying that the child shouldn't be permitted to run naked as a jaybird. I couldn't see what the problem was. After all, the child was still wearing his skin, and his spirit was still in his body. Even at that young age, I realized that I was living in my human body for now, but there was so much more to my existence.

Spiritual integration with the body is very important. It can bring about accord between the frequency of the Fifth-Plane soul and the frequency of the Third-Plane body without sacrificing abilities. One way to help this process is clearing negativity in the body through belief work.

I believe that babies are aware of every emotion around them. In the past, scientists believed that babies couldn't see until they were a month old, but mothers have always known that their baby could see them from the first. Now science is going back on what it first believed. This is why they call it science. A scientist is a seeker of physical truth with the right to change their mind! Seekers of perceived truth and – oops, I got it wrong! But everything considered, science has been a good thing, because it encourages intellectual development.

Every one of us has come through a spiritual portal to get to this plane. Many children of the masters have forgotten who they were before they came here and have to be awakened. But masters who come here can naturally awaken to their abilities. It is their divine mission to bring Fifth-Plane consciousness to this plane of existence. This is why it's important to integrate the physical and soul essences through the higher self.

DIVINE CONSCIOUSNESS: THE HIGHER SELF

The higher self is the supreme spiritual essence that is in all living beings. It is the divine connection to the subconscious mind. It helps us become aware of our divine attributes and gives us guidance on changing undesirable attributes. In some people, it is a means of intuitively speaking with animals, small children, and people who are unconscious or in a coma.

The higher self has an intimate knowledge of the workings of the soul. It is closely connected to that microcosmic dimension in our space where the larger part of the soul resides. It has knowledge of the soul's divine timing. It is our connection to the God-self that is developing in all of us. It is has more of our Fifth-Plane self in it. This soul energy is very powerful and it is important to send the consciousness beyond the confines of it to free ourselves from the belief systems that may interfere with communicating with the Creator.

However, although the higher self is wiser than the mental and physical ego, it still has its own ego, and opinions that may not always be for the highest and best. For this reason, you should always go up to the Creator of All That Is, who has complete understanding of everything. This is where the highest truth resides.

Talk to Your Higher Self

Seen intuitively, the higher self appears as a royal essence just outside the body, connected to the pulsating soul energy between the crown chakra and the top of the head. It has a direct connection to the soul along an etheric pathway that connects the soul to the Seventh Plane of Existence.

So the higher self is outside the human body, yet it is inside the aura, the bubble of energy that in most people extends about three feet around and six feet above the body. It is important to go through the aura when doing readings, because it can be easy to confuse the higher self and the All That Is energy.

When I do readings on myself, I make sure I project my consciousness out of my paradigm to the Seventh Plane for a second and then come back and look into the body. This way I get the view from the Creator's perspective rather than that of my higher self. Then I ask the Creator to show me what needs to be done in my body.

It's the same when I work on others: I go up out of my paradigm so I can heal from the Creator. If I only went out of my body as far as my higher self, my perceptions would only be as divine as my higher self was able to be.

Ask yourself this: do you understand the difference between talking to your higher self and talking to the Creator? Although your higher self is a higher aspect of you, it isn't all-pervasive in and of itself, as the Creator is. The Creator has no ego and is perfect truth.

TALKING TO THE HIGHER SELF

This exercise is designed to teach you the difference between talking to your higher self (or the higher self of a client) and the Creator of All That Is.

1. Go up to the Seventh Plane (see pages 13 and 14) and make the command: 'Creator of All That Is, it is commanded to speak with [individual's name]'s higher self. Thank you. It is done. It is done. It is done.'

2. Go into their heart chakra. Travel upward from their crown until the higher self is found.

3. Speak to their higher self and then tell them what you hear.

4. Rinse yourself off with Seventh-Plane energy and stay connected to it.

I've taught thousands of students and I can generally tell if someone is doing a reading from their higher self or from the Creator. I can tell by the energy in the tone of their voice. When they start getting nervous, the information can be coming from their higher self instead of the Creator. The reason for this is because they aren't maintaining a pure Theta wave and need proper discernment.

When asked a question, the higher self will likely connect to group consciousness or come up with its own opinion before it asks the Creator, unless it is trained to do otherwise. For example, if I were to go up to my higher self and ask who the next President of the United States was going to be, I would find my higher self saying, 'This world is corrupt, the government is corrupt, and you have no say in who's going to win the election, so why are you asking?' But if you go to the All That Is, you get the absolute truth.

When I went up and asked the Creator who was going to win the 2000 Presidential election between George Bush and Al Gore, the Creator told me, 'Vianna, stay focused on your life. Pay attention to where you are. Love the people around you, make a difference in your life and work on *yourself*. If you do this, you'll be able to help others.'

'Okay, Creator, but who's going to win the election?'

'Vianna, stay focused on yourself. It doesn't really matter. There won't be a clear winner of the election and no one will know who wins for weeks after, and it won't be the one who wins the popular vote.'

God was right. There was a recount that lasted for weeks.

The way that we train the higher self to connect to the Creator is to go consciously to the Seventh Plane on a daily basis. In this way the subconscious mind learns to live life with the divine energy of the Creator.

Belief Work and the Higher Self

When you start changing your beliefs, you start bringing more of the higher aspects of yourself into your body. The more virtues you acquire, the more your higher self comes into your space. But if you are angry and resentful all the time, less of your higher self is within your space. Someone like the Dalai Lama, for instance, has many aspects of his higher self within his space.

The only way that the higher self can stay in the human body, though, is if negative beliefs are cleared. Clearing beliefs helps you to become healthier, stronger, and more like your God-self. As you begin to expand psychically, it is imperative that you change your negative beliefs at the same time, in order to keep your body at the same vibrational level as your spirit.

It is difficult to keep the vibration of the higher self in the body, because it can drain the body physically. To have more of your higher self without draining your physical body, go up to All That Is more often. This will balance the body.

INTEGRATE THE HIGHER SELF INTO THE BODY

Virtues required: Helpfulness, honesty, kindness, loyalty, nobility, and trustworthiness.

Integrating the higher self into the body can help the soul essence understand the physical essence so that the two can work together toward common goals.

The more beliefs you clear, the more integration there will be between your higher self and your body, and the healthier you will become.

1. Go up to the Seventh Plane (*see pages 13 and 14*) and make the command: *'Creator of All That Is, I command [or request] to integrate my higher self with my physical body as much as possible, making my body strong and bringing it into my space now. Thank you. It is done, it is done, it is done.'*

2. Witness the higher self coming into the body through the crown chakra and integrating with it on a cellular level in an amazing energy of love, gentleness, and strength. Only let enough of the higher self into the body to strengthen it.

3. Once you choose to break contact, disconnect by rinsing yourself off in Seventh-Plane energy and stay connected to it.

Your higher self is sensitive to your experiences, but whether you have a good experience or a bad experience is immaterial to it, since, after all, it is not material. From the perspective of the soul, you can learn and grow just as easily from a bad experience as you can from a good experience. On a higher spiritual level, if we have learned something from an experience, then it was of benefit to us. The trick is to make it a positive experience. From the Seventh Plane it's possible to create whatever experience you wish to have on this Earth.

The Divine Mission of the Higher Self

One of the higher self's functions is to acquire virtues so that the soul can learn, expand and grow. It is useful to talk to the higher self to find out what virtues are needed.

Vianna: Do I have permission to speak with your higher self to ask which virtues it needs to acquire?

Rose: *Yes, I give you permission.*

Vianna: When I connected to your higher self, it handed me a list written in cursive in red and black ink. The first item was '*Service.*' The second was '*Learn to let someone love you completely and learn to love someone completely.*'

This was written in black ink: 'You have already learned how to be humble. You have also learned how to be brave. Two weeks ago you learned how to appreciate all the good things that you have done in your life.'

Rose, your higher self says that you get annoyed with stupid people, but you're learning to have patience with this planet and mostly with yourself. These are the most prevalent things that you're working on at this time.

What virtues does your higher self need to acquire?

DISCOVER THE DIVINE MISSION OF YOUR HIGHER SELF

Our higher self has its own mission statement and knows the virtues that it has learned and those that it needs to learn.

1. Pair up with another person and talk to each other's higher self to find out the virtues it is learning and those it needs to learn.

2. Then go up to get the perspective of the Creator to see what downloads are needed.

This process should only take five minutes or so.

THIRD-PLANE INSTINCTS

Animal Instinct

Every animal on this planet is equipped with the intelligence that we call instinct. For some reason we humans think that instinct is a lesser form of intelligence than the conscious messages the body sends to the brain. What most of us don't know is that it runs our lives more than we realize.

The trick is to be aware of our instincts and utilize them for our benefit. This is one of the reasons why we learn to do a body scan on ourselves, as explained in my first book, *ThetaHealing*. The body scan gives us direct information about what is happening inside our own body. Who knows, you just might save your own life once you get to know your physical body through intuitive perception.

We have the same kind of instincts as animals, however latent or forgotten they may be. For instance, the police say things like 'I had a gut feeling' or 'I just knew he had a gun – I could sense it.' This is fine, but you cross the line when you say, 'I psychically saw he had a gun.' That's the same thing, but to many people the word 'psychic' has negative connotations. This attitude causes us to be blind to the psychic side of human instinct and may also be why we don't consider how psychic other animals are.

Every species of animal has developed psychic senses in order to survive, and we have done the same. When a woman first nurses her baby, for example, there's an immediate communication without words. Then the woman's body creates antibodies in the breastmilk to meet the ever-changing needs of the child. To me, this is spontaneous intelligence of the human body that supersedes rational thought. In fact, rational thought is useless in some survival situations.

But there are other ways in which the human body communicates with other humans without the conscious mind knowing it is happening, and this is with the reflexive process of pheromones.

Animal Attraction

Pheromones are chemicals that we secrete in our sweat and other bodily fluids as messengers. Most of us automatically change the smell we give off every time we are sexually attracted to someone in the hope that they will be drawn to our fragrance. But what is amazing is that in many instances these responses occur without conscious thought. This means that we can be attracted to another person through smell and from this smell get an instinctual understanding of the messages that are in their DNA!

Some scientists think that we are attracted to one another more by smell than by looks. So we are charmed by a *subconscious* interpretation of someone's energy. But if we were to become *consciously* aware of what we were smelling, we'd be able to understand that person in a profound way. We could smell if they had a disease, or a genetic defect, or were mentally unstable. If we could perceive smells as a dog does, we could psychically identify these secretions.

What is the sense of smell? When you smell someone else, you're sensing particles, atoms. DNA is floating into your nose to stimulate you in such a way to instinctually create a response. This is itself is a form of language, since information is exchanged. When your body accesses this information, it has a good idea if the person is sexually compatible with you or if they have enough in common with you for you to get on with them. This may be why you're attracted to a particular type of person, since your DNA is reading theirs for compatibilities on all levels – mentally, spiritually, emotionally, and physically – through the chemical message of smell.

I believe that the process of procreation uses the best of the DNA material it is given. This means that certain physical and emotional attributes are sent on in the fusion of genetic material for the benefit of humanity.

Some people I've talked to tell me that they are not only sexually attracted to another person's body, but to an inexplicable essence they can't explain. I think that some people are attracted to a vibration that is a little higher than their own. This goes beyond being attracted by smell and into the realm of spiritual attraction.

If you meet someone and are attracted to them, there's a change in you on all levels, from your smell to your attitude. Have you ever wondered how married partners know that their spouse is sexually attracted to someone else? It's because their scent changes, as do their energy and body language. This is all happening on a genetic level. Women suddenly become nicer, because men like women who are nice. Men immediately make more semen to fight off the semen of other men. All of these things happen instinctively.

The Autonomic Nervous System

Another good example of an instinctive reaction that is working in our body is the autonomic nervous system, a network of nerve fibers that regulates the iris of the eye and the smooth-muscle action of the heart, blood vessels, glands, lungs, stomach, colon, bladder, and other visceral organs, all without the conscious intervention of the higher brain centers. However, because it is linked to the other systems of the body, the autonomic system is influenced by the emotions; for example, anger can increase the rate of heartbeat, fear can cause a fluttering in the stomach, and contentment can bring down the blood pressure. How does it know how to do this?

Researchers believe that the human mind, together with the physical body, generates an electromagnetic field of energy. We know that the human nervous system uses what could be considered an electrical current to send vital information throughout the body for a variety of life functions, from computing sensory information to the organization of cellular chemistry and firing electrons across the neuronal synapses. The body itself is obviously electromagnetic, consisting of charged particles such as atoms, electrons, protons, and ions.

All life-forms on the planet consist of subatomic particles moving at different frequencies. Every life-form vibrates at a different pace, but we are all made up of arrangements of particles. In the end, we are only particles moving at slower and quicker paces. This movement results in energy signatures being given off in the form of light, sound, and electromagnetic fields, and these are a means of communication. I believe that all animals, including humans, have their own special ways of communication that go beyond the normal senses and function without conscious thought.

DNA Intuition

Another system of the body that works without conscious thought is DNA. This is the program that is secretly running everything in our body, though we are unaware of it.

Every animal on this planet has been able to modify its intuition to help its survival and it is the same with us. We always want to take ourselves out of the animal world, but we are animals nonetheless. We are mammals and have children that we protect fiercely. Why do we bother to protect them? We know instinctually that they are the future. This instinct was passed down to us from our ancestors. Can we physically define this attribute? Where does it come from? Where is it in the body? It is in our DNA.

Our DNA is constantly creating intuitive survival mechanisms and is working for us more than it is working against us. For instance, even if you've never seen a snake before, it's likely that you'll instinctually feel fear when you do see one. This reflexive instinct stems from DNA knowledge.

Our DNA can feed data into a network, just as we can with the internet. If it can also call up data from this network and establish contact with other participants on the network, then we may have an unknown connection with people who share our direct DNA, such as relatives.

This vein of thought can explain part of remote healing, telepathy, and remote sensing. It may also be why some people can sense their relatives feeling pain when they are miles apart.

If we take this concept one step further, we can say that we share DNA with every other human on this planet and to some extent with every other animal. This means that it might be possible to connect to the DNA in others. This would explain group consciousness and hyper-communication. It would also explain how we can retrieve the ancestral memories and past lives of other people.

REMEMBERING ANOTHER PERSON'S PAST LIVES

In this exercise you will do a reading on a person and remember their past lives or ancestral memories. There is no division between the past, present, and future, since all three are happening simultaneously. Thought and consciousness move faster than the speed of light and as such are outside the Law of Time. By using a condensed lite thought-form, it's possible to bend the Laws of the Sixth Plane and go forward in time then back in time to experience someone else's past life by remembering it as you would when you remember the future. This teaches us that there's no such thing as linear time in a three-dimensional universe.

When you witness a person's past life, focus on the positive aspects and not upon the negative.

1. Go up to the Seventh Plane of Existence (*see pages 13 and 14*) and make the command: *'Creator of All That Is, it is commanded [or requested] that I see and remember [name of person]'s past life now. Thank you. It is done, it is done, it is done.'*

2. Witness yourself going forward in time and then backward into the person's past life. Observe silently and remember. Ask, 'The last time this happened, what could they have done to make things better?'

3. Tell the person all the good things about this life experience and focus on the positive things that were learned from it.

4. Rinse yourself off with Seventh-Plane energy and stay connected to it.

THIRD-PLANE ANIMALS

If we can connect with other people through our DNA, what of the animals with whom we share the Third Plane?

In ancient times our connection to animals was one of a hunter-gatherer symbiosis. This turned into a wholesale domestication of select species that were of obvious benefit to our survival. Hunter-gatherers eventually became herdsmen, and animal husbandry and agriculture were born. This was the dawn of domestication and a different kind of symbiotic relationship that exists to this day. Humans began to enslave other humans and other animals too. For the past 10,000 years, we have genetically altered domesticated animals to suit our needs and have unfortunately driven some into extinction.

More recently, however, there has been a resurgence in the concept of an interconnectedness with all things, including animals. The relatively new science of DNA has shown us that we share much of our biological make-up with the other animals of this precious world. The way that the DNA is structured might be different in each species, but the foundation remains the same in all, including humans. This suggests that we have common origins, no matter where and how these came into being. Whether we humans evolved on this world along with our brother and sister animals or we came as starseeds from another place is ultimately irrelevant considering that while we might be different on the outside, we are much the same on the inside.

It is wrong for people to think that an animal is less intelligent or less intuitive because its brain is smaller. We have a huge brain and we only use a small portion of it. Animals have smaller brains but might utilize their brain tissue in such a way that size does not matter.

Do animals have souls? Of course they do. Do they progress through the planes by transmigration of their soul energy? Of course they progress, just as we do.

This 'new' philosophy of the interconnectedness of all living creatures is not actually new in any way. In India it has been taught for thousands of years and has flowered into vegetarianism. On the other side of the world, Native Americans considered that all life was part of one great whole and animals were equal to humans. Some Native Americans were hunter-gatherers who killed and ate animals, but they were taught to respect and thank the spirit of the animals they killed. In fact, the first 'gods' of many of the tribes seem to have been councils of animals.

Early belief systems in many areas of the globe postulated that humanity was a part of the scheme of things and not in any way superior to other species. To native peoples, everything on this planet is connected, from the smallest crystal to the largest whale in the ocean. But in order to understand how interconnected everything is, we must go on an exploration of how we interact with other animals.

Healing Animals (The Non-Human Variety)

Some of the best friends that many of us have are our pets. They are the very essence of unconditional love.

The way we pick our pets could be the same as how we pick our mates. If we're afraid to be loved, we'll pick a pet that is a little standoffish and distant. If we're a nervous mess, our pet is likely to be a nervous mess. The animal reflects our energy back at us.

Somewhere in the middle of thousands of readings with clients who had pets, I came to the realization that if the pet was sick, so was the master, and vice versa. If I did a healing on the master, then we did a healing on the pet. If it was the pet that was sick, it was imperative that we did a healing on the master. I knew I needed to investigate this phenomenon.

The sickest person that I ever saw in my life had Lyme disease, histoplasmosis (fungus in the lungs), cancer, and encephalitis, and that was just for starters. What I found strange was that her cat was just as sick as she was.

At first I thought that her cat was actually giving her some of the diseases that developed over the time that we worked together. But when I went up to look at the situation from the Seventh-Plane perspective, I found that it was the other way around.

Most pet cats think that they are human and grant their masters the privilege of having them as a pet. But this cat was different. She was compassionate and really loved my client. She was trying to heal her and as a consequence becoming sick herself.

It was very strange, because there were many times when my client would come close to death, only to have the cat take on the sickness. Each time my client would get a little better, but the cat eventually died in this cat-and-mouse game of healing.

This was when I began noticing a recurring behavior with animals. Whenever people came to me and asked me to heal their dog, I'd check to see what the dog was taking from them in the way of physical or emotional distress. Sure enough, if the client had diabetes, the dog would die of diabetes.

I realized that dogs and cats had been bred for specific traits and duties, and over the centuries, some had developed the talent of healing their masters. This had then been passed down through the DNA.

As I investigated this phenomenon I realized the pets didn't have the ability to get rid of the sickness they'd taken on. They would keep it unless I pulled it from their master. The best results came when I worked on the master, then the pet.

Connecting with Animals

I discovered that the healing worked better if I asked the animal's higher self for permission to do it, because animals can't communicate in words.

If the higher self says 'no' to healing, we can reason with it, but should respect the decision.

In many instances, an owner will attempt to make their pet live when the pet wants to die. The owner will psychically hook the animal and make it live. The animal loves the owner so much it will try to live. But we should go up and ask what the higher self wants to do, just as we would with humans. We should ask the spirit if it would like to stay or go.

I also found that an animal will sometimes have core beliefs that need to be removed and replaced and will even need feelings instilled such as 'I know what it feels like to receive and accept love.'

All these elements came together to form the healing protocol I use with animals.

First of all, you should introduce yourself to the animal. When doing this, you should expand into the animal both psychically and physically and give it your sacred name. The animal now has a DNA imprint of you and this lets it know if you are harmful or not. Even when working on an animal remotely, I always introduce myself first.

Then ask the animal for its sacred name. Every animal has one. It can be a tone, an energy signature, or a name. The animal will give you it as an imprint, a vibration that might be heard as a slight sound.

TALK TO AN ANIMAL'S HIGHER SELF AND ASK FOR ITS SACRED NAME

1. Go up to the Seventh Plane (see pages 13 and 14) and make the command: 'Creator of All That Is, I command [or request] to meet the higher self of this animal now. Thank you. It is done. It is done. It is done.'

2. The higher self of an animal can often be found floating above the animal. Go to the higher self of the animal and ask for its sacred name.

3. Wait for the vibration that is the name.

4. As soon as the process is finished, rinse yourself off with Seventh-Plane energy and stay connected to it.

When you 'go in' to speak with an animal, you need to realize that most animals do not understand the spoken word. A much more realistic way to communicate with an animal is to form a picture and then telepathically transfer it to its mind. Most animals communicate by sending pictures and vibrations. They do not intuitively send words, but use feelings, emotions, and images.

It is also very important to understand that sending a feeling is very different to sending words. You are sending an emotion to the animal. So, if you find yourself in a situation where you feel threatened by an animal, don't project the thought, *Don't bite me.* Projecting any kind of image about biting may be misinterpreted and you could cause a biting incident. Instead, project pure love to the animal and move away when you can. In some situations, it may be best to stand your ground, but this is not always the case. Also bear in mind that sending a projection of love telepathically won't work on all animals. Discretion is definitely the better part of valor when it comes to dealing with animals.

SENDING A PROJECTION OF AN IMAGE
OR EMOTION TO AN ANIMAL

1. Go up to the Seventh Plane (*see pages 13 and 14*) and make the command: *'Creator of All That Is, it is commanded [or requested] to send a projection or emotion to this animal. Thank you. It is done, it is done, it is done.'*

2. As soon as the process is finished, rinse yourself off with Seventh-Plane energy and stay connected to it.

Animals can become chronically depressed, just like humans. If you have an animal who is depressed and lethargic, you should project a mental picture to it that it is in a happy situation with its master as its friend, giving it love.

Another way of connecting with animals is to put your hands on them and psychically retrieve information from them. It will likely be in the form of pictures of what the animal has experienced. I suggest that you practice this form of body scan a few times so that you are comfortable working on animals.

BODY SCAN AN ANIMAL

Make your every movement full of confidence and strength while psychically projecting the same feelings.

1. Go up to the Seventh Plane (see pages 13 and 14) and make the command: 'Creator of All That Is, I command [or request] to meet the higher self of this animal now. Thank you. It is done. It is done. It is done.'

2. Ask the animal's higher self for permission to do a reading.

3. Then ask the animal its sacred name and wait for the vibration that is the name.

4. Scan the animal and, if needed, witness a healing or send any negative energy to God's light (see below, page 170).

5. To send an image of love and happiness to an animal, command that a projection of happiness and love be sent to it.

6. Bring yourself up and out of the animal's space.

7. Rinse yourself off with Seventh-Plane energy and stay connected to it.

Animals feel pain with an incredible intensity that can make it difficult to work with them. It may be necessary to relieve their pain before witnessing the healing. Another tool is to go in and project the feeling of the animal being strong and healthy.

Belief and Feeling Work on Animals

Animals usually respond to healings quickly, but if they don't, they may need belief or feeling work. They benefit from belief work that changes genetic programs and core belief programs. Go up and ask their higher self permission to do healings and belief work on them.

Some of the feelings that animals may need are:

'I understand what it *feels like* to receive and accept love.'

'I know what it *feels like* to be loved.'

'I know what it *feels like* to be important.'

'I know how to live without feeling abandoned.'

BELIEF AND FEELING WORK WITH AN ANIMAL

Virtues required: Acceptance, compassion, courage, faith, forgiveness, gratitude, hope, kindness, restraint, service, and wonder.

1. Go up to the Seventh Plane (*see pages 13 and 14*) and make the command: *'Creator of All That Is, I command to meet the higher self of this animal now. Thank you. It is done, it is done, it is done.'*

2. Ask the animal's higher self for permission to do belief work on it.

3. If it is given, talk to the higher self and ask the animal its sacred name. Wait for the vibration that is the name.

4. Get permission for each belief that is removed and replaced and each feeling that is downloaded.

5. Witness the beliefs and feelings being replaced and downloaded.

6. Bring yourself up and out of the animal's space. As soon as the process is finished, rinse yourself off with Seventh-Plane energy and stay connected to it.

SEVEN PLANES OF EXISTENCE

Clearing Negativity

Animals respond quickly to healings, but you may want to work on the owners as well, given that an animal often absorbs sickness from its owner. This is why it is very important to clear your pet of negative energy on a regular basis.

CLEARING AN ANIMAL OF NEGATIVE INFLUENCES

To clear an animal of negative energy, simply seek its permission then go up to the Seventh Plane and command that the energy be gone. Just as when working with humans, you may want to bring the DNA of a very strong ancestor forward when you work on an animal. Witness the diseases or emotions being released from the animal and sent to God's light.

1. Go up to the Seventh Plane (see pages 13 and 14) and make the command: 'Creator of All That Is, it is commanded [or requested] to speak with [animal's name]'s higher self. Thank you. It is done, it is done, it is done.'

2. Ask the animal's higher self its sacred name and wait for the vibration that is the name.

3. Then ask if the animal would like a clearing of the negative energy it has collected from its master.

4. Once you have permission, witness the Creator clearing the animal of negativity.

5. As soon as the process is finished, rinse yourself off with Seventh-Plane energy and stay connected to it.

Animals are so sensitive that you should never put your animal in the same room with people who are sick. Unless you clear them afterwards, they will pick up negativity. This should be an example for us as well. There are times when we take on negative influences without knowing we're doing it.

Emotional Trauma in Animals

It is obvious that when animals are with an owner who is calm, they feel relaxed as well. This is particularly true of dogs. It is important that pet owners realize that their pet is feeling their feelings. If the owner is stressed, the pet takes these feelings as its own in an attempt to clear its master.

If an animal has been abused in the past, the energy of the abuse will be evident in its behavior through emotional imprinting. If you find an animal that has been abandoned, you may find that it needs to clear this trauma. In both these cases, use belief work, just as you would with a human. You can either work through the animal's higher self, just as you would with a human child, or you can connect to the animal and energy test yourself as a proxy for it. Once you find the memories and beliefs that are causing the animal to act out, remove them and replace them with good ones.

The World of Dogs

How fast does ThetaHealing work on animals? Unbelievably fast! This is because some of them in particular are hyper-tuned to psychic vibrations as well as having a range of other senses. Dogs are a good example.

I have a Maltese dog. The Maltese is one of the oldest breeds, with a verified time-span of 2,800 years and a conjectured one of over 8,000 years. There is evidence that it came from Asia to the isle of Malta and was then disseminated through the rest of the known world. Originally used for hunting, over time it was trained to taste the food of the aristocracy to guard against poison and bred as a comfort dog. In Europe it came to be called the sleeve dog because it was carried in people's sleeves. Intuitively, you can touch these dogs and see the generations of kings and queens who were their owners, and see the dogs themselves working as a sort of high blood-pressure medicine.

Seen psychically, my dog, Jasmine, has a white energy that at first seemed like snow. She also had a little fragrance around her so we called her Jasmine after the white jasmine flower. When she and I touch each other, there is an exchange of DNA knowledge that connects us on an instinctual level.

How deep does your consciousness go into someone's space when you shake their hand? What can you pick up? Can you match the intuitive ability of a dog?

When most dogs come into contact with you and lick your hand, they can read what is going on in your body and in your life. They can see if you are fearful or calm, if you are stressed or if you need love. Then they will begin to release pheromones to heal and comfort you.

If your dog can read your DNA through taste, think what kind of knowledge it gets when it smells you! A dog's sense of smell may be 100 times better than a human's. You've watched dogs sniff each other's hind-ends? They're getting a DNA imprint that gives them a complete record of the other dog. The strongest DNA imprints come from the lips, the mouth, and the other, less savory orifices!

I know that every time Jasmine licks me or smells me she's shifting gears to comfort me. She changes her heartbeat, her pheromones, and her healing energy in order to raise my mood.

Dogs have such a heightened sense of perception that they're used for people with special needs – they are trained to help people who are blind, people who have diabetes and people who suffer from seizures. They are sensitive to their master's every move, both mentally and physically. They can hear changes in their very heartbeat. We are blessed to have these special animals sharing our lives.

Horses

The modern domesticated horse has had a relationship with humans for an estimated 6,000 years. In the modern world there are all kinds of horses with different temperaments – some good, some not so good. Some horses get very attached to their masters, much like dogs. Again like dogs, they can sense when their masters are insecure.

When working with horses, bear in mind that they are sensitive around their ears and don't like them to be touched, but once they trust you, they like to have their ears scratched. When you walk around a horse, you need to keep one hand on its back as you walk behind it so that it knows that it's you there. This is a safety action to ensure that the horse doesn't kick out at you, as it would with a predator.

Everything that horses do is down to the fact that predators have hunted them for millions of years. Because of this they are always on the alert and can even feel, from the vibrations of the earth, when you're walking up to them. A horse can feel you long before you get there, so when you first walk up to it you should move in a way that tells it that you are present but not a threat. A horse can sense through the vibrations of your movements if you are furtive, fearful, or predatory. Unless it has been trained not to respond to the smell of fear that you exude, it will be ready to run.

Horses use their legs to communicate with the world, so this is what you use to get to know them. Most horses will become calm if you work with their legs. The more you're able to touch a horse's legs, the more it trusts you, so if you own a horse, it's best to clean its hooves yourself.

Now let's psychically experience a horse first hand.

CONNECTING WITH A HORSE

1. Walk up to a horse projecting confidence and strength, not submissiveness. There is a happy medium between being over-assertive and under-assertive.

   If you walk up and mount the horse without introducing yourself, it won't get to know you in the right way. If you walk up to it and meet it the way it's used to being greeted, it'll remember you forever and respect you. Even when working on a horse remotely, I always introduce myself to it first.

2. Introduce yourself both psychically and physically to the horse by blowing in its nose (both sides, because this is what happens when a horse meets another horse). This tells the horse that you're worthy of its respect by projecting strength and security through the pheromones that you're sending out in your breath. It's important that you witness these feelings and emotions being sent to the horse through your pheromones as well as psychically.

   In just one or two seconds, this exchange of DNA will have told the horse if you're secure or strong or weak and fearful. A horse knows very quickly if you're going to be friends with it or not.

3. Give the horse your sacred name and ask for its name. What will it do in response? It'll blow back into your face and tell you its name!

4. Start walking around the horse with confidence, while psychically projecting the same. Every vibration your feet make will be felt by the horse. If you're tense, the horse will sense it. Be relaxed and calm.

   If you're a little nervous and unsure when you approach a horse, these may be its feelings, not your feelings. Once you are aware of this, you can calm it down.

   As you walk around the horse, put your hand on its back so it knows where you are at all times and feels safe.

The key is to identify with the horse. With its permission, you're going to expand into it to feel what it's like to be a horse.

EXPAND INTO AN ANIMAL

With the permission of the animal's higher self, you're going to expand into it to feel what it would be like to be that animal. You will feel its legs, feel its body, and feel it move. That way, you will get a DNA imprint of what it feels like to be the animal.

1. Go up to the Seventh Plane (see pages 13 and 14), become comfortable and take a deep breath in.

2. Imagine that you and the animal have become as one on a molecular level. Feel what it is like to be the animal. Move as the animal, think like the animal, get a DNA imprint of the animal. Your molecules and those of the animal are transferring back and forth. The two of you are connecting, becoming one.

3. When you have finished, rinse yourself off with Seventh-Plane energy and stay connected to it.

The Aura of a Horse

The aura color of a horse will tell you volumes about it.

FIND THE AURA COLOR OF AN ANIMAL

1. Go up to the Seventh Plane (*see pages 13 and 14*) and make the command: *'Creator of All That Is, it is commanded [or requested] that I see the aura color of this animal. Thank you. It is done, it is done, it is done.'*

2. Witness the aura color of the animal.

3. When you have finished, rinse yourself off with Seventh-Plane energy and stay connected to it.

What do the colors mean?

- White means a perfect demeanor and great healing abilities.

- White or green sparkles mean healing energy.

- Blue means the horse is extremely sensitive and does not respond to force. It also means it is attempting to read you. A gentle voice will calm it down.

- Red means that the horse is fearful and sees danger everywhere. It is timid and defiant at the same time and will respond if you witness white light expanding into it.

- Gray means that the horse has worms or is sick.

- Purple means the horse is jumpy and trusts only a few people. It will be responsive to Seventh-Plane energy.

SEEING A HORSE'S AURA

1. As you walk around a horse, notice the color of its aura. This will change in different areas of its body. If it is startled, the color will flare for a second and then return to normal.

2. When you first touch the horse, go up to the Seventh Plane of Existence and imagine it turning to pure light… What color is it? Imagine merging with it.

When I watched the movie *Ladyhawke*, I was fascinated by the black horse that they were riding. I found out that it was a Friesian and it became my dream to own one. The Friesian line comes from the Netherlands and was originally bred to carry knights into battle. Later, Friesians became dressage horses, carriage horses, and light draft horses.

Recently I had the opportunity to own one of these majestic horses and I got Feja. She is a mare whose bloodline comes from the Netherlands. The first time I touched her, I went into her space and her aura appeared as sparkly white energy. I think that this was because when I touched her I went up to the Seventh Plane and she was instinctively matching that color and energy.

I learned something new from Feja when I took her to the ThetaHealing Institute of Knowledge so that my students could experience what it felt like to go into the space of a large animal.

I noticed that each time a student touched Feja, her aura color changed to whatever aura color the student was emanating at the time. Her emotional state changed too. If the person was nervous, Feja was nervous. If the person was calm, Feja was calm.

I feel that this is a form of communication that only special animals have: they give us back the energy we emanate and magnify it.

The Mystical Cat

There are two types of cat: cats who get attached to their environment and cats who think they're human and get attached to their owner. Those who think they're human are the ones who possess mystical qualities. They act as natural psychic energy enhancers for their owners.

Our pets are a mirror of who we are, a mirror of our very soul, and this is particularly true of cats. They magnify whatever energy their owner projects, either good or bad. A cat can give energy, magnify energy, or take energy.

Mystics used cats as energy magnifiers in their workings with the divine. Cats enhance many different psychic abilities, such as telepathy and the clairaudient, clairvoyant, empathic and prophetic senses that we all use to some extent.

Cats heal their owners when they are sick and can also work as energy enhancers when the owner does healings on others.

Animals that are similar to the cat in that they act as energy enhancers are crows, ravens, most raptors, and some smaller dogs, though most dogs have more of a give-and-take friendship with their owners. Most human–cat relationships are those where the cat permits the human to have it as a pet.

Most cats choose their owners. They pick someone they can communicate with telepathically when they choose to. Most owners don't even realize that they're telepathically communicating with their cat.

However, there are cats that aren't really cats at all but something different. Some are spiritual energies (living in a cat) that work as guides to help people find their life path.

When you psychically talk to a cat, it's a good idea to do so through its higher self. It will become agitated if you go into its space without talking to its higher self first.

Animals in the Wild

The 'Animal Problem'

I've always had what I call an 'animal problem,' ranging from large animals to very small ones: animals are somehow unaware of me and, even when they're in close proximity to me, fail to see me. This happens mostly with wild animals, because dogs, cats, and horses have always seen me just fine, and most have loved me. But with wild animals, as I've explained in other books, it's as if I'm invisible to them.

After reflecting on why this is happening, I've realized that I don't give off the DNA vibration of any kind of a threat and the animals perceive me as either a plant or a smaller animal. This has been to my advantage in that it has permitted me to get close to wild animals.

This was demonstrated when I went to Australia for the first time.

Animals of Australia

Before I went to Australia I wanted to see a koala in the wild because I knew there was something special about them. I put my request in to God a week before I went, so there was plenty of time for it to be processed. But when I arrived in Australia, the Aussies told me that koalas were rarely seen in the wild and never came down from the trees.

Our seminar was staged at a large house in the mountains above Coolangatta on the Gold Coast. The conference room had no air-conditioning and during the lunch break Guy and I took a stroll to the forest to get out of the heat. There we noticed a koala bear had crawled down a tree right in front of a car. It was moving along very slowly and precisely, and as we watched it, it climbed up another tree. I was so excited to see it in the wild!

When I went back to the class, the students told me how very rare it was to see koalas in that area. But when I'd put in my request to the Creator, I'd believed I'd see one, and life is all about belief.

In Idaho I lived in a place where there were houses all around me and I constantly attracted families of moose into my yard. I knew they were around when I perceived their light ballerina-type energy.

I even attracted a gray wolf to my back door. One night, I felt compelled to look out the tempered glass of my door and when I did, I locked eyes with a wolf that was staring right at me.

The point is, if animals know they're safe, they'll show themselves to you. Of course I realize that you probably don't want to attract certain animals. So you should send the manifestation out to the universe to bring the animals you want to see and not those you want to avoid.

Connecting with Wild Animals

Before you come into contact with wild animals, you should probably do some belief-work sessions about how you feel about them. Energy test for 'I'm afraid of wild animals.'

If you were born with a fear of an animal, use the fear digging work to find the bottom belief that's causing it. I've worked with several people in India who were born terrified of tigers. I had to go back into different lifetime energies to clear their fear.

It's best to have common sense with animals of any kind and follow the safety criteria set down by park rangers and other knowledgeable naturalists. Wild animals (particularly large carnivores) are best seen from a distance. This is why God helped us to create binoculars and wide-angle lens cameras!

When you're walking through the wilderness, you should put out the signal that it's safe to do so and everything around you is safe. This way, you're going to see a lot more animals without being hurt by them. It is particularly important that this signal of safety is sent out when you run into an animal. Instead of sending out a signal of fear, keep sending, 'I am safe.' It is also best to do your research and follow the guidelines of experts on wildlife in the area.

I strongly suggest that to connect with the wild animal kingdom you expand your consciousness into an animal (*see page 174*). Try it with a spider first. Spiders are very psychic intuitive creatures and if you send them the thought that they should leave your house, many times they will leave. They won't argue as much as you might think.

If you practice this technique with animals in the big national parks, you'll find that wild animals are much more tuned into you than you may realize. When I go to Yellowstone Park, I usually go up and ask the Creator to show me a particular animal.

Good luck on your animal healing journey!

DUALITY AND DRAMA

It can be easy to get obsessed by the duality and drama of the Third Plane, especially when contemplating aliens, UFOs, metaphysics, and conspiracy theories. Clear answers are hard to come by, though certainly there are aliens out in the universe who are thousands of years beyond us in technical development. We have a lot of catching up to do to be on a par with some of these races.

It's interesting that technological development was once very slow on Earth. For instance, the Iron Age began around 1200BCE but didn't reach its full potential until the advent of the blast furnace in the 1600s. It took over 2,000 years just to find a reliable way to make cast iron and steel. But after the Second World War we started developing faster than at any time in recorded history. Why did this happen? Did we get information we'd never had before? I don't like to dwell on these things, but I've had some very strange experiences...

Something weird was happening in Idaho Falls in 1996 and 1997, something beyond anything that I'd ever experienced before. The first thing I noticed was bizarre alien phenomena with psychically inclined women who came in for readings. I worked with these women and they generally got better. Word spread and it wasn't long before a fair number of people were coming to my office complaining of alien implants in their body or visitations from aliens. Since I had no fear of this kind of thing, I simply removed the implants and sent them to God's light. Some of these people became lasting friends of mine.

Then I began to notice a pattern to these strange occurrences: many of these people worked at the Idaho National Engineering Laboratory, the nuclear site outside Idaho Falls.

One man, who told me he worked for NASA, had what looked like seven foreign objects in his body. This was the most I'd ever seen. I asked myself, 'Are these actually alien implants, or has he created them with his mind? Does he believe in the existence of these implants so much that he's actually created them?'

Setting aside my belief systems and doubts, I focused on what would benefit my client. I went up and asked God to get rid of the implants and watched as they were removed in sequence: first from the neck, then the spine, then the ankles. The man thanked me and left.

After that, female clients began to come in who were five months pregnant. The health of mother and fetus would be fine, but a few weeks later the women would be back distraught: the baby had simply vanished. I was told that there had been no discharge and I knew that the body had not absorbed the baby, since the pregnancy was at an advanced stage. Each of these women had had an ultrasound as proof that it wasn't a false pregnancy. The baby had simply vanished overnight.

When I asked the Creator what was happening, I was shown the strangest thing: someone from the future had come and taken the babies. They were safe, but they were somewhere in the future where the human race had become sterile. I saw that on some level the future selves of these women had made an agreement with their past selves in this time. I don't know how this had happened, but I could sense that the babies were fine and the women would get pregnant again soon.

I would chalk these occurrences up and put them on my 'unexplainable' shelf. I knew that the nuclear plant did some secret experiments and perhaps this was why some people in our area had UFO experiences.

I asked the Creator, 'Why do people see UFOs and claim to be abducted? Are aliens among us?' This is the information I received.

First, every speck of sand on the planet has memories of everything that has happened here. All the events are recorded in the Earth itself. Our bodies are made of the same essences that are in the Earth. Our bones are made of the minerals of the periodic table. This makes the human body a memory-keeper too.

Secondly, I was shown that in the distant past an advanced race came from the stars and seeded humans on this planet. We are seeds from the stars and the DNA starseed that is inside us has affiliations with many planets in this universe. This planet itself has had many civilizations.

Thirdly, I was shown that there are memories in the light that shines down on Earth. This means that the entire universe has memories of everything that has happened in it. These memories may be the reason why intuitive people sometimes get the feeling that they are from other planets.

Then I saw the ascended masters returning to this planet to inhabit human bodies, bringing their experiences from other places and planets in the universe.

I was also shown people contacting aliens from other planets with the power of their thoughts. I was told there were many worlds in the universe with life on them.

The first time I went to England, Guy and I were walking through Glastonbury when I looked across the street into the eyes of a being that I was sure was a gray.

One other thing I'm sure of: not all the people who told me they'd had 'alien experiences' had actually been abducted or even contacted by aliens. Some of these people used the alien experience to cover up molestation experiences. But there were some alien experiences that were completely unexplainable and they happened to rational scientists in high-paying government jobs.

There are many theories about reptilians and grays, and it may be that there are aliens traveling through space by folding a time continuum. I have memories from a time in ancient Egypt when people walked in through doors that folded time. I was one of them. We came from Arcturus on a mission to teach healing, farming, and other practices. I'm uncertain where this memory comes from and it isn't really important. All that matters to me is that healing knowledge came forth into this life.

There are things out there that are difficult to explain, but the main thing is not to permit the fear of these strange occurrences to overwhelm us and deter us from our divine timing. What is important is the energy of pure thought and love.

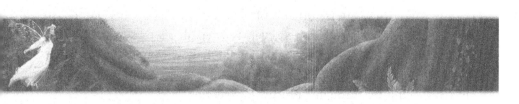

7

THE SECOND PLANE OF EXISTENCE

The molecular structure of the Second Plane of Existence contains a carbon molecule and is therefore organic matter. So this plane consists of plants, trees, and elementals and it teaches us to be in harmony with them. Within this harmony, we learn the first lesson of how to use light energy to heal.

This chapter is dedicated to the secret intuitive world of plants and trees and how they relate to our existence on the Third Plane. It looks in depth at how to communicate with the plant kingdom and gives an explanation of the much-misunderstood elementals that some people call fairies. Much of the information here has been written for some time and was sprinkled through my earlier books. But when I started this book, new information began to come in. There was so much information on trees, plants, and animals that I decided to create separate classes on the secret lives of plants.

SYMBIOSIS WITH THE SECOND PLANE OF EXISTENCE

For thousands of years, trees, plants, and humans have developed an interdependent relationship. Plants use humans to propagate and spread, and in turn they are indispensable to human survival and the foundation of civilized society.

This symbiosis is not unique to plants and humans. The relationship between plants and insects is undoubtedly much older than the one that we now enjoy. Bees are the friends of plants, but grasshoppers and locusts are perhaps not. So plants have developed repellents to deter unfriendly insects and fragrances to attract friendly ones for pollination. These strategies may be, as scientists say, a process of evolution, but we have been able to speed it up through a process of selection.

Archeologists think that the cereal plants that we now call wheat and barley were developed in the 'fertile crescent' of the Middle East in the last 10,000 or so years. They were once simple grass plants growing wild that were selected over other plants for their qualities as food. The selective breeding process undoubtedly took a long time, but now these plants are the staples that give us our daily bread. Other grains and vegetables have also undergone slow genetic alterations over thousands of years of development, at least until recently.

Vines, bushes, and trees that had small insignificant fruits in their original wild state have also evolved through selective breeding to culminate in the cornucopia of grapes, apples, pears, cherries, bananas, and plums we know today.

Learning how to cultivate and rotate crops must have been a rather difficult trial-and-error odyssey that probably spanned many generations. But once this simple process was learned, it gave us a survival tool more effective than any before or since: a reliable, renewable source of food. This was the dawn of civilization as we now know it.

With the spread of agriculture, we began to alter the very landscape to suit our survival needs. Three simple plants enabled us to change the face of the world: wheat, oats, and barley. Where great forests once covered the landscape, there are now farmland and cities. This process continues today in places like South America.

Most of the foods we now consume have a long history of selective symbiosis with us. The question is, who is using whom? Are these plants using us as part of some grand ecological survival plan, or are we the masters?

Time will tell how effective a survival tool the relatively young technology of agriculture will be in the next 20 years of population growth and genetic modification.

ENLIGHTENED BEINGS

I once asked the Creator to introduce me to one of the most enlightened beings on Earth. I was surprised to be taken to meet a tree. I watched it go through its life processes: it used water and minerals from the soil and light from the sun in the process of photosynthesis, the sacred transformation of blessed sunlight into pure energy. So I realized that trees and plants were some of the most evolved of God's creatures, acting out the sacred dance of connection between the Second and Third Planes of Existence.

Trees and plants transmute the sacred life-force so that animals can utilize it. They gather nutrients from Mother Earth through their roots and long after they die they continue to return those nutrients. They follow Nature's sacred cycle and only compete to live, not to destroy. While only consuming sunlight and air and using the soil to sustain themselves, they provide nourishment and shelter for all other living beings.

The actual life-force, the *light* that is within the tree or plant, is important to the human body. It is through utilization of this light that we stay connected to all the planes of existence. Most creatures of the Earth need sunlight to live. It is the essence of life itself. Everything on this planet is based upon the fire of light.

A good example of how plants use light is photosynthesis, which is a process in which the energy in sunlight is absorbed by the plant, converted into glucose and stored for the plant's later use.

WITNESS PHOTOSYNTHESIS IN A PLANT OR TREE

1. Go up to the Seventh Plane of Existence (*see pages 13 and 14*) and make the command: *'Creator of All That Is, it is commanded [or requested] to see photosynthesis in this plant or tree. Show me. Thank you. It is done, it is done, it is done.'*

2. Go to the plant or tree as gently as a feather on a summer breeze. Imagine the light being processed by the plant or tree and turned into sugars.

3. Rinse yourself off with Seventh-Plane energy and stay connected to it.

In the process of photosynthesis, plants *absorb* light to create energy. But I believe that they use light in the opposite way as well. I believe that they can *exude* it in subtle ways in order to communicate with one another.

PLANT COMMUNICATION
Gently, Softly

One day I was listening to some tapes I'd recorded years ago for some of my earlier manuals. It was beautiful, interesting information. However, what I found truly fascinating was that the essence of the vibration I'd been then was very different to what it is now. The way I've communicated my essence to the world has changed over the years, as has my vibration. Now my essence is much smoother and more compatible with my environment. The way that I psychically communicate with the world has changed as well. I'm very gentle in the way that I communicate with the human body.

It is very important to be gentle while doing a body scan so that the immune system doesn't thinks you're a foreign invader. It's important to witness a healing with gentleness as well.

Much of this approach to energy healing was learned by psychically experiencing trees and plants. I found I had to be very gentle when I went inside them with my consciousness.

SCAN A PLANT

This exercise is designed to introduce you to the Second Plane, to demonstrate how sensitive plants are, to teach you how to move in and out of their living space, and to allow you to practice your scanning abilities. This will sharpen your skills as well as your discernment.

The way to scan a plant or tree is to introduce yourself and go into the plant, be there for five seconds or fewer, and come out of its space. This way the plant has the full signature of your thought-forms and you have the signature thought of the plant. This is the beginning of communication between you.

Be gentle throughout the process: plants and trees are very sensitive and if you push your thoughts toward a plant too forcefully, it can literally die.

Virtues required: Compassion, creativity, forgiveness, gentleness, safety, and understanding.

1. Go up to the Seventh Plane of Existence (*see pages 13 and 14*) and make the command: *'Creator of All That Is, I command [or request] to scan this plant. Show me what I need to see. Thank you. It is done, it is done, it is done.'*

2. Go to the plant as gently as a feather on a summer breeze. Now imagine going gently into the plant, taking a quick look and then taking yourself out of its space. Remember, if you go in with too much force, you can actually harm the plant.

3. Rinse yourself off with Seventh-Plane energy and stay connected to it.

Talking to Plants and Trees

As I scanned plants and trees and started to get information, I realized that there was a lot I didn't know about them. At first I didn't know how to talk to them. Plants communicate in several ways:

- *Through light.* The most important way that trees and plants communicate is by using light to talk to one another.

- *Through the roots via the soil.* Plants and trees communicate through their roots by sending subtle vibrational messages using the minerals in the soil. In more advanced trees, the roots are connected to another tree and communicate directly.

- *Through chemicals.* A plant or tree exudes these chemical messages with the intention of reaching other plants in the area as well as repelling or attracting insects.

These are languages that we can train ourselves to understand. We can convert them into tones or pictures and then convert these into words.

Why do we learn to talk to plants? Dualism is a pervading essence of the Second Plane of Existence. From it, we learn that for every poisonous plant there is an antidote plant. This is why we talk to the plants. All plants have a great purpose in the grand scheme of things.

A polite way to address a tree or plant is to ask its name and tone. Everything in nature has its own special way of greeting and every plant has a sacred name.

Many of us are too busy and loud with our thoughts to even hear plants and trees. Again, gentleness is the way to connect to them.

LEARN THE LANGUAGE OF PLANTS AND TREES

1. Go up to the Seventh Plane of Existence (*see pages 13 and 14*) and make the command: *'Creator of All That Is, it is commanded [or requested] that I learn the language of this plant or tree. Download the feeling and knowing of its language and show me. Thank you. It is done, it is done, it is done.'*

2. Witness the feeling and knowing of the language of the plant or tree being brought into you on all levels.

3. Rinse yourself off with Seventh-Plane energy and stay connected to it.

When you've mastered talking to plants, each and every plant can tell you if it is beneficial or poisonous.

It's not uncommon for a tree to attempt to find out what your motives are before it permits you to talk to it. It will explore you first. For instance, I went to the Sequoia National Park once to talk to the giant trees that were there. What I found was that the redwoods would talk to me openly, but when I went into a sequoia's space, it treated me almost as if I was an ant, saying, 'What do you want?'

'I am a human,' I told it. 'I want to talk to you.'

'I don't think so.'

I tried again: 'No, really, I want to talk to you.'

After attempting to talk to six of them, I finally found one who would speak with me. He told me about his long life growing in the forest. This helped me to realize that each tree had its own personality.

In another encounter with trees, I went to the forest behind my former home to listen to the cottonwoods there. I found that each of them would speak to me in a friendly way.

COMMUNICATE WITH A PLANT OR TREE

1. Go up to the Seventh Plane of Existence (*see pages 13 and 14*) and make the command: *'Creator of All That Is, it is commanded [or requested] that I communicate with this plant or tree. Show me. Thank you. It is done, it is done, it is done.'*

2. Go to the plant as gently as a feather on a summer breeze. Now, imagine going gently into the plant or tree and asking it for its sacred name.

3. Give the plant feelings of gentle love and say its name (silently) as you communicate with it. Give it your sacred name so that it will become comfortable with you.

4. Rinse yourself off with Seventh-Plane energy and stay connected to it.

As I investigated plants and trees, I saw that they communicated with one another to an amazing extent. A tree that is being attacked is able to broadcast a warning to other trees in the area. If the attack is from insects or fungus, this gives the other trees time to formulate chemicals against them. If a tree or plant is healthy, it can fight off insects, fungi, bacteria, and viruses.

Plants and trees have thought processes and soul energy that are peculiar to them. They are aware of light signals in a way that we are not. Animals and humans emit light signals and never realize that plants and trees are intimately aware of these emissions. They know when we walk past them.

Trees are highly evolved organisms. Some groups of trees are actually one giant organism. A good example of this is the Pando, also known as the trembling giant. This is a massive interconnected group of quaking aspen in Utah. This colony – a huge clone – encompasses 106 acres (43 hectares) and has around 47,000 stems, which continually die and are renewed by the roots. The root system is among the oldest known organisms – it is an estimated 80,000 years old – and the aspen colony communicates through it.

While some trees communicate through the root systems, others, with shallower root systems, use different forms of communication. For instance, lodgepole pines in Yellowstone Park communicate through light and sending chemical messages through the air. Although conifers also communicate using their roots, they are not as effective at it as other species.

Many species of plant and tree are highly intelligent and pick up the essence of our thoughts. Thoughts move faster than the speed of light and we are very loud in our thinking. Trees actually have to protect themselves from our loud thoughts in order to stay centered. They are aware of us as we walk in the forest and can perceive if we are friend or foe.

If they feel there is a predator around, plants and trees can change their chemical structure. The different species of plants in our garden will alert one another in this way. They act as one entity when a message of danger is sent out.

Trees and plants that bear fruit expect the fruit to be eaten. That is how they procreate. It's why there are seeds inside our fruit and vegetables. But when root crops are pulled from the ground and eaten, this causes the plant distress. This is why it is so important to bless a plant as you harvest it, so that its spiritual essence goes swiftly back to the light. This is an important cycle that is also a kind of spiritual symbiosis.

Nowadays we are very selective in the plants and trees we consider valuable. In the past, other trees and plants were our choice. It's freakish to see psychically how some of these react to our presence both negatively and positively by communicating whether we're a threat or not.

Grasses

Grasses don't communicate in such an intricate way as trees, but do realize when an animal is grazing on them and use their shallow root system to transfer this information to other grasses. They can also protect other grasses by making themselves less palatable to the predator.

Even if they are eaten, most grasses can grow back very quickly, as cropping causes their roots to spread beneath the ground. They have also learned to use animals in a symbiotic relationship. The plants know that the animal will spread their seeds and pollen so that they have a better chance of survival, and when they are fully seeded, they actually signal to animals: 'Come and eat me!' so that their seeds can be spread. Once the animal defecates with the seeds intact, the feces act as fertilizer for new growth. This symbiosis has likely been going on for millions of years.

WITNESS PLANTS AND TREES COMMUNICATING WITH ONE ANOTHER

1. Go up to the Seventh Plane of Existence (*see pages 13 and 14*) and make the command: *'Creator of All That Is, it is commanded [or requested] that I witness this plant or tree communicating with another through its roots, through chemical messengers, or through light. Show me. Thank you. It is done, it is done, it is done.'*

2. Go to the plant or tree as gently as a feather on a summer breeze.

3. Witness it communicating with other plants or trees.

4. Rinse yourself off with Seventh-Plane energy and stay connected to it.

Father and Mother Trees

For every group of trees there is a father and a mother tree. The mother tree is usually much larger than the other trees. She assesses the gossip that is going on in the group to ascertain what the information means. She sends messages of encouragement to the other trees and tells trees of all types what kinds of chemicals to exude to stop attacks from insects, fungi, bacteria, and viruses. She also gives comfort and advice to all her trees.

The father tree has a very protective energy. He will also gather information of all kinds from other trees and plants (not of the same species) for the common good of his group. This includes information on the changing conditions in the soil and in the weather. He also takes in knowledge of the surrounding land and learns how to deal with all the different threats in the area.

Even when hundreds of people and animals are in the mountains, the trees know where each individual is and the father and mother trees gauge the behavior of each one.

If the father or mother tree is killed, another is assigned to take its place. If part of the father or mother tree is damaged, it becomes what is called a grandfather/grandmother tree, a stronger tree is chosen to lead and the ancient knowledge is transferred to it. Similarly, when a father or mother tree becomes too old to continue that role, it transfers its knowledge to a younger tree that assumes the role as leader of the trees.

The problem with our forest service is that it cuts trees down at random, killing the old trees that once led the other trees. This causes a problem for the entire species, making it weaker and more susceptible to disease and predators. With so many old trees being cut down, invaluable knowledge is being lost. Stopping the over-harvesting of old trees is a good plan.

MEET THE FATHER AND MOTHER TREES

In this exercise it is best to learn the language of the species of tree that you are going to meet, then introduce yourself and let the father and mother trees scan you. After that, you can converse with them. Trees are very wise in all matters and can give you good advice. They may need help from you in some way as well.

1. Go up to the Seventh Plane of Existence (*see pages 13 and 14*) and make the command: '*Creator of All That Is, it is commanded [or requested] to see the father and mother trees of [area]. Show me what I need to see. Thank you. It is done, it is done, it is done.*'

2. Go to the trees as gently as a feather on a summer breeze and introduce yourself with your sacred name.

3. Allow them to introduce themselves with their sacred names.

4. Now imagine going gently into either the father or mother tree, taking a quick look, and then taking yourself out of its space. If you go in with too much force, the tree will reject you and won't talk to you.

5. Rinse yourself off with Seventh-Plane energy but stay connected to it.

PLANT HEALING
Plants and Vibrations

Plants and trees are designed to absorb light, water and nutrients, and minerals from the soil. These all have a beneficial effect on them, but what about substances that aren't beneficial?

Plants also absorb pollution from the air, the water, and the soil. A plant can absorb strychnine, mercury, lead, and other negative chemicals and still grow, but when it or its fruit is harvested and eaten, these chemicals go right into our systems. This is why juicing our vegetables is so important, since many of these chemicals stay in the pulp and aren't in the juice. Carrots, beets, and celery are good choices.

Another good example of the ability of plants to absorb negative substances is when herbicides are used to kill them. Herbicides are designed to work as systemics, meaning the chemicals are absorbed by the whole plant, even the roots. But again, eventually, the heavy metals make their way back into our own systems too.

In addition, plants and trees absorb electromagnetic energy and radiation of all kinds. Today we send radio waves through the air and communicate using cell phones. Cell phones give off radio-frequency (RF) waves, which are a form of non-ionizing radiation. In most of the studies that scientists have undertaken into cell phones, there has been no conclusive evidence that they cause health risks. However, one study did find that while using a cell phone for 50 minutes, the body used more glucose than normal. This may be one reason why I feel that radio frequencies affect plants in adverse ways, since they use glucose to survive.

We have created cell-phone towers that employ energy and have failed to realize that these emissions can damage plants and trees. I believe that plants and trees are so sensitive to these energies that they are weakened by them and fall prey to infectious and parasitical diseases as a result. This is because these energies disrupt their ability to communicate through light.

Those who think that the thoughts of other people have no effect on our body and mind should consider all the electrical waves, radio waves, microwaves, and other forms of radiation to which we are subjected and the effect these have on us and the world around us. When you consider that the brain is an electrical generator, it's obvious that the combined thoughts of a million people will have an effect. Since it's difficult to measure the electrical energy of millions of people, a scientific study on this has never been done. But this doesn't mean that this kind of electrical energy doesn't exist or have an effect of some kind. And if a large majority of these thoughts are negative, what kind of an effect will they have, especially on highly sensitive plants and trees?

This is why we should send positive energy to plants and trees. They are highly intelligent in their own way and will eventually adjust to the new radio waves, given time and support.

We should also realize that if these waves affect plants, they must affect us as well. We would be wise to keep cell-phone radiation out of our houses. Of course we still want to use our cell phones, so commanding and witnessing that all excess radiation that our cell phone emits is sent away from us is also a good plan. We can use the Seventh Plane to command that we are impervious to radiation, use common sense to keep cell phones away from our sleeping areas and command the extra radiation to go to the light. We can also do this for our own plants, gardens, and trees. Because we are part of a Fifth-Plane presence, we are unbelievably powerful and can send this excess radiation back up though a portal to be changed and used as pure energy.

Commanding and downloading that the plants know how to adjust to RF waves is also good. If a plant is given good soil, plenty of sunlight and the proper nutrients and taught how to adjust to radio waves, it will become healthy and strong and will be able to fight off any attackers that come its way.

SHOW A PLANT OR TREE HOW TO ADJUST TO RADIO WAVES

1. Go up to the Seventh Plane of Existence (*see pages 13 and 14*) and make the command: *'Creator of All That Is, it is commanded [or requested] that this plant [or tree] knows how to adjust to radio frequencies created by humans. Show the plant. Thank you. It is done. It is done. It is done.'*

2. Go to the plant or tree as gently as a feather on a summer breeze and witness its vibration adjusting to radio frequencies.

3. Once you have finished, rinse yourself off with Seventh-Plane energy and stay connected to it.

Heal a Plant

If a plant is sick, we can heal it with the help of its sacred name and unconditional love. Using the name assists in the healing because it gives us a reference point to work from.

WITNESS A HEALING ON A PLANT

1. Go up to the Seventh Plane of Existence (*see pages 13 and 14*) and make the command: *'Creator of All That Is, it is commanded [or requested] that this plant [or tree] [give name] be healed. Thank you. It is done, it is done, it is done.'*

2. Go into the plant or tree as gently as a feather on a summer breeze and witness the Creator healing it.

3. Once you have finished, rinse yourself off with Seventh-Plane energy and stay connected to it.

WITNESS UNCONDITIONAL LOVE AROUND A PLANT OR TREE

1. Go up to the Seventh Plane of Existence (*see pages 13 and 14*) and make the command: '*Creator of All That Is, it is commanded [or requested] to surround this plant [or tree] with unconditional love. Thank you. It is done, it is done, it is done.*'

2. Go to the plant or tree as gently as a feather on a summer breeze. Witness the love of creation surrounding it.

3. Rinse yourself off with Seventh-Plane energy and stay connected to it.

Healing from Plants

'Under the branches of the oak, near the trunk, people laid their sick, hoping for help from the gods. Beneath the oak boughs, wives joined hand in hand around its girth, hoping to have beautiful children. Up among its leafy branches the new babies lay, before they were found in the cradle by the other children. To make a young child grow up to be strong and healthy, mothers drew them through a split sapling or young tree. Even more wonderful, as medicine for the country itself, the oak had power to heal. The new land sometimes suffered from disease called the val [or fall]. When sick with the val, the ground sunk. Then people, houses, churches, barns and cattle all went down, out of sight, and were lost forever, in a flood of water.'

FROM *DUTCH FAIRY TALES FOR YOUNG FOLKS* BY WILLIAM ELLIOT GRIFFIS

Have you ever wondered why there is a movement in industrialized nations toward bringing nature back to the cities? There are of course the obvious benefits of air purification. Every day, plants and trees heal us with the oxygen they release. But they also heal us through the vibrations they emit. The song of leaves rustling on the wind, the shade that trees provide and the love that they give are immeasurable gifts if we but take the time to notice.

ACCEPT HEALING FROM A PLANT

1. Go up to the Seventh Plane of Existence (*see pages 13 and 14*) and make the command: *'Creator of All That Is, it is commanded [or requested] that I permit a healing from this plant or tree. Thank you. It is done, it is done, it is done.'*

2. Go into the plant or tree as gently as a feather on a summer breeze and witness it healing you through the Creator.

3. As soon as the process is finished, rinse yourself off in Seventh-Plane energy and keep that energy within yourself.

Healing the Soil and Preparing the Garden

Everyone should have a garden so that they know where their food comes from. The ultimate goal is to use the pure food of the All That Is essence and create your nutrients from the divine, but in the meantime the more organic food you eat, the better. The title 'organic' not only means that the producer is doing their best to create a product that is pure, but that pesticides from nearby fields haven't contaminated the soil in which it has grown.

In the process of developing a garden, preparing good soil is all-important. In modern times we've farmed a great many of the natural nutrients out of our soils and modern farming practices only give the plants three nutrients in the fertilization process. They used to have access to many more.

Another concern we should have is that all the cars and airplanes that drive and fly by our crops leave a residue of fuel that seeps into the plants and into the soil. As we have discussed, plants are designed to absorb light, water, and fertilizers, and they absorb chemicals of all kinds just as readily.

The only way to clean up the soil is to use the same process that is used on the human body: give it the right vitamins and minerals to pull the toxins out. Fertilizers and a balance of minerals will do this in most cases. It is important that you perceive the soil as a living thing that you are healing.

You may wish to put ionic colloidal minerals (trace minerals) into the soil. There are formulas available that are made from a plant source. These can be used in the garden and for any plant or tree that is food-bearing. Plain yogurt gives the soil the bacteria that it needs and adds good humus. Extra natural fertilizers are also a must. If you can find it, wood ash is an excellent addition to your fertilizer mixture. Putting the mixture on at the end of the growing season is best. The soil needs to set over the winter with this mixture tilled into it before you plant in the spring (if possible).

Plants that are grown in this kind of garden will be strong and able to resist the extra radio waves and most other predators that come at them.

In any garden, it is best to avoid the use of chemical poisons in the form of pesticides. If you do use these substances, make sure the residue is washed out of the plants before they are eaten.

Plants compete for space, but even when you pull out weeds in the garden you should make sure that their energy goes to the light. Create the feeling of love around the plant and this will help it grow much better. You can do this with the soil too.

WITNESS UNCONDITIONAL LOVE BEING SENT INTO LIVING SOIL

1. Go up to the Seventh Plane of Existence (*see pages 13 and 14*) and make the command: 'Creator of All That Is, it is commanded [or requested] that unconditional love is sent to this soil that will nurture the plants and trees. Thank you. It is done, it is done, it is done.'

2. Witness the love of creation being infused into the soil. Witness the soil come awake and alive.

3. Rinse yourself off with Seventh-Plane energy and stay connected to it.

Always bless your garden and work in it in a positive way, with excitement and love instead of a feeling of drudgery. Thoughts, both negative and positive, affect the way plants grow. There are many fertilizers that you can use in a garden, but without the basic minerals and thoughts of love, the plants won't be receiving the same essence of light from you, and the light that you eat when the plants are harvested won't be of the highest form.

HARVESTING PLANTS

Love, joy, happiness, and respect are the keys to truly understanding plants and trees. As you harvest a plant, be connected to the Creator, go back to the time when the plant was a seed, pour love and blessings into it, and watch it grow into its present form. This will give it more potency.

HARVESTING A PLANT OR TREE

1. Go up to the Seventh Plane of Existence (*see pages 13 and 14*) and make the request: *'Creator of All That Is, I ask this plant's permission to harvest it. Thank you. It is done, it is done, it is done.'*

2. Go to the plant or tree as gently as a feather on a summer breeze. Speak to it in its language. Witness going back to the time when it was a seed and pour love and blessing into it as you watch it grow into its present form.

3. Rinse yourself off with Seventh-Plane energy and stay connected to it.

The Energy of Food

The food we consume is a marriage of the minerals of the First Plane, the plant life of the Second Plane, and the proteins of the Third Plane. This marriage of the planes is the staff of life, an incredible fusion of energies that brings nourishment to the body. This is why it is important that we eat food that has life in it, such as fresh fruit, vegetables, and wholegrains, without sacrificing any of the proteins that are so important to our body. Think about it – DNA is made of proteins, so what do we need to repair DNA? Proteins!

Some plants are very high in proteins. Wheat, avocados, and soy are some of them, but I feel that we need to be careful about the consumption of soy because a lot of it is genetically altered and may cause cancer. Non-genetically altered soy is best. If you use it, be sure to bless it. Since everything has a consciousness and we absorb this essence when we consume it, we need to bless all the food we eat. Genetically altered food, especially corn, has a consciousness that is perhaps not for our best. If there is a question about the essence of the food, go back and bless it from its origin.

If you buy herbs, vitamins, or food from the store, ask the Creator if they are for your highest and best. You can determine this by connecting to the Creator while holding the product and simply asking if the potency is correct. Once the substance has passed the test, it should be blessed before use to insure maximum potency, effectiveness, and quality.

Even if you have only a window box, you should consider growing herbs. They not only provide nutrition for the body, but also for the soul, as they absorb negativity and change it to positive energy.

Vitamins symbolically give us the feeling of being loved. If they are missing from our food or the body isn't absorbing them, this results in the feeling of a lack of love in the body. Yeast and bacteria, which also reside on the Second Plane, occur naturally in the body, being neither good nor bad. However, it is important that they are balanced in the body. To experience harmony with the Second Plane of Existence, the body must be in balance.

While I think that it's possible to 'psychically' create some of the vitamins and minerals that we get from food, it's also important to realize that our food brings us many benefits that aren't at first apparent. The act of eating and digesting gives us a subconscious understanding of the first three planes of existence and a glimmering of the others. What is important is to be consciously aware of the story that our food has to tell us.

There is an incredible amount of psychic information locked within our food. Through food, we connect with the energies around us and are in constant communication with everything that has ever existed on the first three planes. Once we open ourselves to the possibility, there's almost limitless information in a simple loaf of bread.

We can access the information within food by connecting to the Creator and then going into the DNA to ask what the food is teaching us and is bringing to a conscious level of understanding in us. This simple act of understanding from a DNA standpoint could tell us many things, such as why we crave the food we do. We don't crave anything we don't need, so if you are craving foods that are high in sugar or high in preservatives, you have a lack of something that is in these foods.

With a deeper understanding of food, we would change the way we eat, and if enough people had this understanding, we would change our whole structure of agriculture.

Vegetarians

Many people are becoming vegetarian these days. One reason for this is a concern for sentient beings. This is fine, but plants are sentient too. A carrot isn't going to be happy when you bite it in half.

It's important to understand that everything an animal has experienced is recorded in it. Some of these memories, feelings, and emotions are transferred to the person who eats it, and it is the same with a carrot.

This is why it is best to bless any vegetable or animal protein that you eat and witness the spirit of the plant or the animal being sent to the light. Everything that we eat should be thanked for its sacrifice.

PLANTS AS MEDICINE
The Higher Food: Herbal Medicine

Since the dawn of time humans have used plants in different ways. Herbs were the first medicines and to this day 40 per cent of our pharmaceuticals are made from plant compounds.

Herbs are called the higher food. They have dedicated their existence to medicinal purposes. Herbal medicine can be studied, but if you are wild-crafting (gathering wild plants from nature) the plants for your remedies, it's possible to learn to communicate with the plant itself so that it will tell you if it's friend or foe. You can train yourself to know if a plant is beneficial by touching it and communicating with it. There are many books with pictures for proper plant identification and with practice you'll be able to tell the plants that will heal the body.

When using plants to heal, whether homegrown or wild-crafted from nature, we should remember to harvest them with respect. Through the Creator of All That Is, speak to the plants in their language, express your need and ask their permission to harvest them. They should speak back to you and direct you to those that will best suit your intended use.

There is an organic combination of plants for every illness. But healers using the Second Plane in this way do require an extensive knowledge of herbal remedies and how they work with other medicines. Without this knowledge, there may be a risk to the client. Healing from this plane takes time and persistence.

Herbal remedies should not be taken all the time. Note they are holistic in approach.

'Give Them Light'

We need sunlight, just as plants do, for vitamin D. When we consume plants, we are in a sense eating transformed light.

I believe that the plants that have the highest form of nutritional light are blue-green algae, chlorella, and spirulina. These can revive the entire body. Anytime you get the message, 'Give them light,' you're being told to suggest the use of these plants.

Blue-green algae

Contain biologically active enzymes, glyco-proteins, lipids, minerals, simple carbohydrates, and vitamins. Algae are highly efficient photo-synthesizers and blue-green algae are said to have many health benefits. They are antioxidants and energy boosters, can be used for detoxification, help to balance food cravings, improve memory and mental focus, increase concentration, and pull toxins from the body.

Chlorella

An excellent source of chlorophyll, carbohydrates, vitamin C, vitamin E, and proteins; used for asthma, bleeding gums, burns, and infections; one of the best ways of pulling mercury toxins from the body (must be started with small doses and increased slowly).

Spirulina

A concentrated source of amino acids, chlorophyll, iron, and proteins, it is used to boost the immune system and pull sicknesses and toxins.

Clearing Bad Radiation from the Body

Most people believe that all radiation is bad. But radiation is simply the emission of energy in the form of waves, which includes light. We need radiation to live. In our industrial society, however, we are subjected to an incredible amount of radiation from the wonders of modern technology and I began to notice that the cause of some cancers was radiation. So I began to release the day-to-day radiation of cell phones, computers, fluorescent lights, and other electrical equipment.

To counter the effects of radiation from these and other sources, use the following process. It is best to witness bad radiation leaving the body and good light energy remaining in place.

RELEASING RADIATION

1. Go up to the Seventh Plane of Existence (*see pages 13 and 14*) and make the command: *'Creator of All That Is, it is commanded that all radiation that does not serve [person's name] be pulled, changed, and sent to God's light. Thank you! It is done. It is done. It is done.'*

2. Witness the radiation being pulled and sent to God's light.

3. As soon as the process is finished, rinse yourself off with Seventh-Plane energy and stay connected to it.

Since bad radiation is not a substance that should be in the body, it isn't necessary to replace it with anything.

THE ELEMENTALS

> 'In years long gone, too many for the almanac to tell of, or for clocks
> and watches to measure, millions of good fairies came down from
> the sun and went into the earth. There, they changed themselves
> into roots and leaves, and became trees. There were many kinds
> of these, as they covered the earth, but the pine and birch, ash
> and oak were the chief ones that made Holland. The fairies that
> lived in the trees bore the name of the Moss Maidens or Tree
> "Trintjes," which is the Dutch pet name for Kate, or Katherine.'
> FROM DUTCH FAIRY TALES FOR YOUNG FOLKS BY WILLIAM ELLIOT GRIFFIS

One of the most exciting aspects of the Second Plane of Existence is the elementals, the spirits that guard, protect, and nurture the plant realm. As you experience the plant kingdom, you'll open up to experience them, whether you believe in them or not.

Because of the spiritual evolution and ascension of humankind, the veils are becoming thin between the planes and it's much easier for us to see through them than ever before. The veil between the Second and Third Planes is becoming particularly thin. Because of this, greater numbers of people are witnessing what are called fairies.

I like to call them 'elementals,' and make no mistake, they are not human in any way. Elementals can control the rate of their molecular vibration to merge with plants, become beings of liquid or air, or take a solid form as they choose. It is when they choose to take solid form that we see them in their myriad different shapes and sizes as fairies, because this is the only form that our mind can accept them as.

The Second Plane is the first of the planes that demonstrates the ability to enjoy life and express laughter. It is where we begin to experience diversity in emotions and feelings. This is being learned by the elementals as well. They are also in the process of learning how to make inter-dimensional shifts and to bend time. They are intertwined with the plants, the pure essence of light, and the process of photosynthesis.

The first time I ever saw a fairy, as I related in other books, was when I was with Guy in a cabin the mountains above Sandpoint, Idaho. Guy already knew what they were. He'd worked with the Earth and knew that there were spirits around plants and trees. He also knew about the vast body of ancient lore that centered on the subject.

When I first met Guy, I noticed that when I was around him, he was a walking fairy portal. I think that this was because he understood that the land had an energy all its own and fairies were transmitters of this energy.

That first experience with fairies opened up a whole new realm for me and I realized that fairy energy was centered on plants and trees. Native peoples call this living essence 'the Green.' In European traditions, it's called the Green Man and the Earth Mother, and sometimes there's a fusion of the two aspects. Both can be traced back to the Fairy Queen and the Oak King.

Young Children of the Masters

Everything in the universe uses energy in the highest form that it can, whether it's light from the sun or transformed light created by something else. As we've seen, plants use the light particles they absorb to emit their own light as a form of communication. It is this light that draws the fairies.

Real fairies/elementals shouldn't be confused with modern interpretations of them. They don't always look incredibly beautiful, nor do they always act with benevolence toward us. Though they aren't exactly cute, they are bizarrely interesting. They move faster than the speed of light and generally cannot be seen with the naked eye unless they choose to be seen. We perceive them as having human-like forms, but this doesn't mean this is their true form. Their true form is some kind of spirit light energy.

Elementals may be on the same journey that we embark on through the levels of existence. We leave the Fifth Plane where we were born for the Fourth Plane, the spirit world, where we are tutored, nurtured, loved, and given different assignments according to our abilities. First we are sent to the First Plane to learn the molecular structure of the mineral kingdom and the building blocks of inorganic matter. Once this knowledge has been assimilated, we return to the Fourth Plane to report. Everything we have learned is recorded. Then we are sent to the Second Plane to study the plants. Then we return to the Fourth Plane to report. It may be that young spirits on this early part of their journey are what we perceive as fairies.

Fairy Portals

Elementals are attracted to the light exuded by trees and plants. They help them to grow and send out light to communicate with other plants. They take the commands from the mother and father trees and pass them to all the other trees like a siren. They also use the energy created by trees and plants as portals to other dimensions.

Between mother and father trees there are usually large portal trees that are entranceways for fairies. There are also legends of entranceways in rings of stone and circles of mushrooms. Our ancestors observed these things and didn't fully understand them, but knew they existed. I believe that what many people today perceive as alien visitors are actually fairies using a dimensional portal.

If you can find the mother tree in a forest, look around you. Someplace close is the portal tree. You can take your camera and take pictures of it to capture the energies coming through the portal. You can also do this with a plant.

WITNESS A PLANT OR TREE PORTAL

Virtues required: Adventurousness, hope, kindness, morality, and the ability to manifest dreams and magic.

Blocks: Fear.

1. Go up to the Seventh Plane of Existence (*see pages 13 and 14*) and make the command: *'Creator of All That Is, it is commanded [or requested] that I see the portal of this plant or tree. Thank you. It is done, it is done, it is done.'*

2. Introduce yourself to the plant or tree and go into it and find the dimensional portals.

3. Imagine that the portals are open and that they stay open for a few minutes.

4. Take a picture with a camera.

5. Command (or request) to see fairies and watch the plant or tree become more animated.

6. Once you've finished, rinse yourself off with Seventh-Plane energy and stay connected to it.

When you look at your picture, you'll be able to see small orbs around the plant or tree. These are its thought-forms and the energy field of a portal or the angelic fairies that are around it.

Proper Discernment

Elementals are sometimes afraid of us and won't reveal themselves because they see us as predators. But even if they aren't part of your belief system, the more you're in a Theta state, the higher the possibility that you'll see them with the naked eye. Use proper discernment in working with them, because they're incredibly powerful beings and they don't process thought in the way that we do. They are like yet unlike us.

Fairies are mischievous and extremely curious. They love to annoy us just as much as they love to help us. They are joyful spirits with their own inconsistencies and passions. They're so sensitive to the emotions of humans that they can die from an overload of sadness. They don't like to be ordered around, but can be utilized if approached in the correct fashion.

In one of my classes in Australia, someone came up with an interesting point. They found that anytime they asked the elementals for help, they expected a gift in return. If you find your keys missing from your purse or some other shiny article missing, this can be the fairies exacting their due.

Elementals love shiny things because of the refractive index of light that they create, in much the same way that we appreciate a sparkling diamond. Energy is created when light hits a crystal formation and this luminescence is a divine essence to elementals. This is why they're drawn to crystals. If they're comfortable with you, they'll live in the crystals of your home.

If you decide to open your home up to fairies, or deal with them in any other way, you should do so from the Seventh Plane. That way, the energies of the Second and Third Planes will work together, and human and elemental will enhance each other and not be at odds. If you deal with elementals from a Second-Plane perspective only, there will be an exchange of energy and it's possible that the fairies will take you to another dimension. There are many legends of people being taken by them.

As you open up to experience elementals, here's a list of points to remember:

- Always go to the Seventh Plane before you talk to elementals or go anywhere with them.

- Never ask a favor of an elemental because they expect an exchange of energy, will take shiny objects without permission and feel completely justified in doing so.

- Elementals only show themselves to those who are pure in heart.

- You don't have to believe in elementals to see one.

- They will only show themselves if they know they are in no danger.

- Elementals respect you more if you respect yourself.

- Elementals are not gods.

- Elementals adore laughter and are enchanted by singing (if it's on key).

- Elementals love art. They love watching us paint pictures.

WITNESS AN ELEMENTAL

1. Go up to the Seventh Plane of Existence (*see pages 13 and 14*) and make the command: *'Creator of All That Is, it is commanded [or requested] that I see the elemental of this plant or tree. Thank you. It is done, it is done, it is done.'*

2. Go into the plant or tree and find the elemental.

3. Rinse yourself off with Seventh-Plane energy and stay connected to it.

4. Take a photo (elementals can often be photographed).

Because the veils are beginning to drop between the planes of existence, I believe that some elementals have come to inhabit human form. We've all seen people who act as though they are elves or fairies. It's almost as though they're evolving into fairies or vice versa. I believe that many elementals do this just to have the experience of the Third Plane.

Many of these 'fairy people' are here to protect the elementals and their habitat. They are environmentalists and naturalists.

The Icelandic Elves

The fairy faith is a pre-Christian one that was once held in most of northern Europe. Its roots run deep to a time when we were more in tune with nature and the spiritual energies inherent in it. In places such as Ireland and Iceland, it has survived into modern times.

In Iceland there is a very old tradition of a people called the elves, who are said to live in special places in the landscape. A recent survey has found that only 10 per cent of the Icelandic people believe strongly in elves and other supernatural beings, but road building has been rerouted in order to avoid certain rocks where the fantastic creatures are said to reside.

One of the known elf locations is at Hafnarfjordur, on the outskirts of Reykjavik, where a large rock is said to be an elf habitation. When plans for a nearby road would have destroyed the sanctuary, the road was diverted so as not to disturb the supernatural residents.

About three hours' drive north of Reykjavik, at Ljarskogar, another road was being built when mysterious accidents were reported in front of a stone said to be another haunt of the elves. Work was brought to a standstill while the constructors called in a medium to find out if the elves were to blame for the disruptions. The medium talked to the elves and reported to the workers that the creatures were asking the authorities not to blow their stone up, but to find another way round, so the elf community would not be harmed.

Tourists can find in Iceland a real Elf School, with a curriculum, classrooms, textbooks, diplomas, and ongoing research. There are special textbooks about elves, light-fairies, hidden people, dwarfs, gnomes, and mountain spirits. The materials describe 13 types of elf, three kinds of hidden people, four varieties of gnome, two forms of troll, and three types of fairy.

8

THE COLOSSAL MEMORY-KEEPER, THE UNIVERSE

The First Plane of Existence consists of all inorganic material in the third dimension, all the elements that make up this universe in its raw form, all the solids and almost all the atoms of the periodic table before they start to bind to carbon bases. When carbon molecules are combined with certain elements they form the plant life of the Second Plane of Existence. Then a more complex grouping of molecules is formed that gives movement and mobility. This combination becomes proteins that are the building blocks of the Third Plane of Existence, the place of humans and animals. This is an oversimplification of the incredible process of life.

This material – the living minerals, the crystals, the soil, and the rocks, from the smallest crystal to the largest mountain – forms the building blocks for organic life. Since life begins with these building blocks, it stands to reason that these essences have a spiritual component to them. The First Plane of Existence brings us the realization that inorganic life has life and a consciousness of its own.

MEMORIES IN THE UNIVERSE

Every sun in the universe gives forth light that travels outward. As this light travels across the vast distances of space, it takes on knowledge of everything it experiences and every place it passes thorough. By the time it hits the Earth, it carries with it a host of accumulated knowledge. Every animal, plant, or particle of sand on Earth has the possibility of perceiving all the memories this light has to offer.

Intuitive people are able to perceive some of this knowledge. This may be why people are able to write about other star systems and their ancient cultures without ever having experienced them directly. It may also be why some people have 'alien visitations' that aren't really visitations at all – they are memories carried on the solar winds by the very starlight itself. These two factors could explain why so many people think that they've had a lot of past lives. By just touching or connecting with the Earth or by absorbing starlight, they pick up the memories that are inherent in the universe.

MEMORIES IN THE LAND

Third-Plane beings in turn leave their impressions upon everything they touch, and these are absorbed, as memories, by the First-Plane minerals, soil, and other solid objects. Eventually, they live within the landscape. The memories of every person, animal, and plant that has ever lived on Earth are recorded in every particle of dirt and sand on the planet. If you stop and listen, you can feel the memories that are inherent in the Earth. The most recent are on the surface and are easier to read. In a way, the Earth has its own Akashic Records.

Guy grew up on a farm in Idaho and a ranch in Montana. His great-grandfather, William Stibal, homesteaded the farm in Idaho in the 1890s. At that time the land was wild and had to be settled. William made the ditches for irrigation by following the stars, planted trees, dug a well, put up outbuildings, and built a large house in 1914.

When Guy inherited the Stibal homestead farm 70 years after William's death, the first thing we did was to refurbish the house that William and his son William (Bill) had built. It was a daunting process and it would have been easier (and less expensive) to build a new one. But against all logic, we saved the old house from destruction. During the refurbishing process, I felt compelled to have a stained-glass window installed. Later, I found out that this is what William and his wife, Bessie, had wanted. They had put it in one of the original plans for the house.

Then we put a white fence around the house, just as there had been when William had owned it.

Then we put up a new horse barn and began raising Friesian horses, which are light draft horses. We found out later that William Stibal Senior loved his draft horses and used to pull the tractors out with them when they were stuck. He had a barn that was specifically designed for these horses, complete with sliding windows to feed them from the outside.

Then we had one of the fields leveled, just as he would have wanted.

All these desires had been energetically left there. William's dreams were imprinted on the land.

Sacred Sites

Over time, some sites accumulate their own special energy and are used for ritual purposes. Some examples are the stone circles of Stonehenge and Avebury in England. There are also many Christian churches that were built on ancient ritual centers throughout Europe.

When I first went to Rome, Italy, I stayed in a hotel close to the old Colosseum. When I told my psychic friends where I was staying, they were concerned for me. They thought it must be terrible to be so close to the energy of that awful place! So many people had died there! But I thought the Colosseum was awesome. Sure, lots of people had died there. There was a strong imprint of death, but just as importantly there was an imprint of life, of history, of events that had happened there. I didn't focus on the sadness, but rather on the vitality of the place.

Then we visited Saint Peter's Basilica. This is one of the most beautiful churches in the world. But the person who took me there told me how evil some of the popes were. He asked, 'Can't you feel the evil that pervades this place?'

That wasn't what I was taking from it. It wasn't that I didn't have that feeling, but when you look at the majesty of the artwork there, all that has to take a backseat. When you look at the Pietà sculpture by Michelangelo, you can see how he captured the poignant look on Mary's face as she cradled her crucified son in her arms. Michelangelo also refused to put the imprint of the nails in the hands of Jesus in the sculpture, so that the Son of God would not be flawed by the marks from crucifixion nails. This was because of the love that he felt for Christ, and this love was portrayed in every inch of the sculpture. When you first see the frescos he painted in the Sistine Chapel, you can feel the love that he felt for his work. You can also see his mischievousness – on one wall he portrayed one of the bishops who criticized his work as a demon from hell.

If you look at all the other artwork, you can feel the competition that was going on between the artists as they attempted to finish their work before another artist finished theirs. You could feel the challenge of infusing spiritual energy into every painting and sculpture in the place. But through it all, you could feel the joy of life in those masterpieces.

I felt that Saint Peter had actually been buried on that hill in Rome and that the place had remained sacred in spite of the vicissitudes of evil popes, sadness, and hatred. That sacredness still pervaded the place with a breathtaking resonance.

Some years later I went to a sacred site in Mexico. My representative, Antonio, took me to the shrine of the Virgin of Guadalupe in Mexico City to see the image of the Virgin that had miraculously appeared on a Tilma, a kind of cloak worn by native Mexicans. What I found was that Mexican people came to this shrine to be healed and to renew their faith. Their faith pervaded the place, but there was also some corruption and strange energy in the church.

When I saw the Tilma, I knew it wasn't the original and the real one was behind it, locked away in a room. When I told my guide, he was amazed and asked me, 'How do you know that? I know the security people who protect the shrine and the original is locked away in a vault.'

The point is this: if you look for evil, you can always find it. There is evil in the world, but when people go to sacred places they should enjoy the holiness that pervades them, not concentrate on the negative aspects that exist there. If we focus on the negative, we give it a kind of power that adds to it.

Emotions are very powerful things. If many people project emotions over a period of time in one place, they create energy fields that are stored there. Some sacred sites have accumulated so much energy that they have created bends in time.

Bends in Time

When we die, it leaves a deep impression on the place where it happens. This impression in the land is the reason why psychics sometimes have the feeling that they have to go to faraway lands to collect their soul fragments from past lives. The idea is that once the psychic gathers the soul fragments of their past lives, they also gather the power of their past lives and are complete. This is all based on memories held in the land.

The land keeps the imprinted memory of events of all kinds. The more recent the event, the stronger the emotions and energy associated with it. This makes it easier to see psychically. For instance, in the United States we had a civil war in the 1860s that was the cause of over 5 million deaths. On some of the battlefields of this war, the echoes are very strong, because so much death happened in one place at the same time.

The sudden release of the life-force from the body is an unbelievably powerful action, and when many people die at one time, a vortex of energy forms a large bend or warp in time and a portal is created. This is one reason why some people can see a battle going on even 100 years after it has happened.

This is only one kind of bend in time. There are many different kinds, all with different causes, like the one I found in Yellowstone National Park many years ago.

Yellowstone National Park is one of my favorite places in the world. One of the reasons why I stayed so long in south-eastern Idaho was to be close to it. It's one of my 'power spots,' a special place I go to be recharged by the volcanic energy there. Volcanic energy also creates a bend in time.

The first time I saw the bend in time at Yellowstone was many years ago while walking down one of the trails by Old Faithful geyser. As I crossed a bridge spanning a beautiful river, I saw a Native American couple who were obviously in love with one another. (And no, they weren't doing anything sexual, they were just sitting blissfully enjoying each other's company.) I had a very strong feeling of recognition when I saw the woman and this sparked a strong feeling of *déjà vu*. Many memories began to come back to me about her life and I came to know her as 'She Who Talks to the Wind.'

This is one of the reasons why I like to go back to Yellowstone Park from time to time: to see these two lovers and to get recharged by the energy of this special place.

I've found it's easier to see this divine couple when it's a little foggy or rainy. Why is it that I can see them at all? I think that there are several reasons. I think that I was this Native American woman in a past life and the intense feeling of love between these two people has made an opening in time, but in a different way than a battlefield or a violent death.

I once had a man come in for a reading who had ghostly Native Americans walking through his house. He thought they were wayward spirits, but when I went over to his house to send them to God's light, I perceived that the phenomenon was a bend in time. Because these spirits weren't waywards, I didn't know how to change the situation for him. I told him that it was harmless and that he should charge admission for people to watch it. Had I known what I do today, I would witness the opening of the portal being moved outside the house to another place.

A bend in time is an opening to another time. You can see the people there, but they can't see you. They are living their life, and that moment is what you are seeing in the bend in time.

A Bend in Time from Quartz Crystal

Because quartz crystal magnifies psychic energy, I have many crystals in my house. I have the mineral kyanite as well, so that the energy of the quartz crystals doesn't cause headaches.

In my former home in Labell, Idaho, there was so much energy in the house that a bend in time was created and I would see a ghostly farmer walking through my living room. The farmer was oblivious to my house and thought he was plowing his field, but he was actually in two places at once. He wasn't a ghost and I could only see half of him, because ground level in his time was several feet lower than my living room, so I would see half of him walking through my living-room floor! Admittedly, this didn't happen all of the time, and only when the conditions were right, such as when there had been a lot of rainfall.

There were other times, too, when I saw a Native Indian tepee when I was looking out of my back window across a little bridge that led to a cottonwood forest. This vision wasn't a ghost, but an echo from a different time.

THE MEMORIES IN MOTHER EARTH

Memory-Keepers

Light is the grand accumulator of knowledge and the memories in it are easily stored in the Earth. The minerals of the Earth keep the memories of all the events that have happened in the past. They absorb memories not only from living plants and animals, but also plants and animals that have died and returned to the Earth. Gemstones have the ability to magnify memories in a way that far exceeds that of other minerals. Emeralds, diamonds, rubies, sapphires, and tanzanite are all very good at accumulating both memories from living things and light from the stars. Even though they've been buried in the Earth, they hold the memories of the light of the sun as well as the memories of other suns in the universe. This is one reason why we receive inspiration when we wear crystals.

RETRIEVE PAST KNOWLEDGE FROM A GEMSTONE

1. Go up to the Seventh Plane of Existence (*see pages 13 and 14*) and make the command: *'Creator of All That Is, it is commanded that I retrieve all the past knowledge that is in this stone.'*

2. As soon as the process is finished, rinse yourself off in Seventh-Plane energy and stay connected to it.

Every crystal that is on Earth has some kind of memory within it and as a consequence has developed the ability to accelerate the energy of animals and humans. This is why you can use minerals to enhance your intelligence or improve yourself in another way.

One of the abilities of certain kinds of First-Plane crystals is automatically accelerating the Third-Plane essence of the person who wears them or carries them. This is termed as a marriage of the Third and First Plane of Existence energies, and if you could see this interaction through the eyes of a psychic, the display of energy passing from the stone to the person and back again would be an interesting one.

There are some practical dos and don'ts when handling crystals. You should never place crystals or minerals in water and then drink the water. Some crystals and minerals have toxic substances in them, such as arsenic, lead, cadmium, manganese, iron, and a host of other less than savory substances, and these can leach into the water. If you drink it, heavy metal poisoning will be the result.

Not only can these First-Plane energies accelerate attributes that you already have, but earth essences can also be programmed to complement your life and to work for you. The minerals and crystals that are in your home or work should all be given a specific job to do.

When I first began to do the DNA activation, I programmed a few of my crystals to download the DNA activation into others. When people touched them, their DNA would be activated. This was so that the knowledge would never be lost. You can program a special stone or piece of jewelry to be your memory-keeper.

CREATE A MEMORY-KEEPER

Download your experiences into your record-keeper.

1. Go up to the Seventh Plane of Existence (see pages 13 and 14) and make the command: 'Creator of All That Is, it is commanded [or requested] that I download the knowledge of my experiences into this record-keeper. Surround it with love.'

2. As soon as the process is finished, rinse yourself off in Seventh-Plane energy within yourself.

You can download the crystal with the ability to record what you've learned anytime you touch it. When you travel, program it so that everywhere you go feels like home.

If you program jewelry and it's passed down to your children, it'll have your energy signature and they'll be able to connect to you wherever you are on the planes of existence.

Some of us are still looking for jewelry we had in another life that was charged with ancient memories that we may never find...

Energy Stones

When people in my classes see that I'm wearing beautiful gemstones, they should know that I'm drawn to them because of the energy they emanate as well as their beauty. I rarely buy diamonds, for instance, because I'm just not drawn to them. They don't have the energy I like. I've found that some diamonds need to be cleared of the memories of violence and intrigue that they carry with them. This is why I won't buy blood diamonds.

The following stones are those I've found give me protection and energy and match my vibration. The reader will have to find what kind of stones and minerals are right for them.

Amethyst

Amethyst is the birthstone for February. It is part of the cryptocrystalline family of common quartzite. It is produced when a quartz crystal has a high content of iron in it. This introduction of iron is what causes the deep purple color in the stone. Most amethyst on the market is heat-treated to enhance the color.

Amethyst is one of a family of stones that can be used by the intuitive. The name comes from the Greek, meaning 'not drunken.' Amethyst was considered by the Greeks and Romans to be a strong antidote against drunkenness. It symbolizes sobriety to this day.

A myth of its origin comes from the Greeks. The story goes that Bacchus, the god of wine, was angered by a mortal who refused to recognize him and vowed to vent his fury upon all mortals who didn't participate in his drunken ways.

Amethyst was a beautiful young maiden on her way to worship the goddess Diana when she was detained by the angry god. Bacchus summoned two tigers to devour her, but Amethyst cried out to Diana for help. To save the girl, Diana transformed her into a statue of pure white quartz.

When Bacchus saw the beautiful statue, he was moved to tears and began to weep in sorrow at his actions. His tears fell into his wine goblet and he collapsed, spilling the wine over the statue. The clear white quartz absorbed the color from the wine and the god's tears, and amethyst was created.

As you can see, the energy of amethyst has been popular for thousands of years, and it is one of my favorites. This stone opens the intuitive to the planes of existence. It opens the third eye and the abilities inherent in the crown chakra. When placed on the body, it opens a person to their psychic potential and enhances their healing abilities. Placed in the house as a cluster, it clears and sorts through negative energies that come in through the door or are absorbed through the walls. It is a vital stone to have in your house for this reason.

Andradite Melanite Garnet
This gemstone is one my favorite stones. It can hold energy under a pyramid and it was the first stone to wake up my intuitive senses.

Apophyllite
Apophyllite constantly wakes up the DNA to our divine timing.

Aquamarine
Aquamarine is a stone from the beryl family that healers should have in the home to create comfort and help their connection to heaven and Earth energies and the Creator. This ocean-colored stone works as a psychic bridge because of its association with the energy of water.

Black Onyx and Obsidian
Black onyx and obsidian are both good stones to have to protect against free-floating negative feelings in the home and office.

Celestite
Celestite makes us aware of our spirit guides and angels.

Citrine

Citrine is the yellow-gold variety of quartz and a sister of amethyst. Natural citrine is rare and much of the citrine on the market is heat-treated amethyst or smoky quartz.

The golden color of citrine gives it its ability to trigger abundance and create financial stability, since it is the color of gold. When I'm talking about abundance, I'm not only referring to money, but health, balance in relationships, family abundance, and spiritual abundance. I have a large natural golden citrine that I use to bless my students with abundance.

On a physical level, the stone will help to cleanse the liver and balance the solar plexus chakra.

Spiritually, it brings us to the realization that we can create what we want and integrates our spirituality into our life a common-sense fashion. It magnifies empathy so that we can perceive the feelings of others in a balanced way.

Amethyst and citrine are my favorite crystals to put in the house.

Diamond

Diamond has long been the symbol of love. The stone is a tool of spiritual awakening, but it is not, to my mind, as effective as apophyllite.

Dioptase

More and more people are being drawn to dioptase as a psychic stone because it heals the heart, magnifies the energy of the heart, and brings kindness.

I have some very fine natural specimens of this stone that have the classic emerald-green color with a strong hint of blue. Placing dioptase in your house provides a strong reminder of the attribute of kindness, but, as with all things, it is up to you to accept this strong suggestion from the stone.

Emerald

One of the great planet-healing gemstones on Earth is the emerald. This is the stone that the queens of Egypt wore in the ancient world, and there are reasons for this. In both raw and gem form, this amazing stone of the beryl family has a high frequency of vibration. Real emerald brings back attributes and experiences from past lives and reminds us of everything that we will be in the future. It also brings information from different times and places multi-dimensionally. It brings clarity to any records that have been kept in the metaphysical world.

In its cut gem form, the emerald keeps us calm and aware. When we wear it or put it in our home, it brings forth the best we can be. It magnifies healing of the physical and spiritual body, with an emphasis on helping heart problems.

The emerald is vital in this time of great change. Many ancient records are waiting to be discovered in its heart. Less expensive versions of emerald are now available and a high cost doesn't always mean a gem has better attributes.

Fire Opal

Fire opal is another stone that is important at this time. Since it is a soft stone and is formed primarily from water, it works as a bridge between dimensions, places, and times. It brings back energy that is lost when someone gives too much of themselves to others, and so brings back lost soul shards. It also enhances every spiritual attribute we have and mixes well with other stones, in spite of rumors that it does not.

Gold and Silver

Gold is one of the most important of all the elements in terms of metaphysics. It enhances everything, but also brings the body to perfection. Gold is both male and female, and affects both sexes in the same way, in spite of the tradition of gold being a sun metal (male) and silver being of the moon (female). It should be worn to stay grounded in this reality, but it will also permit us to leave this illusion at will. In this way it helps us reach the spiritual realms and still be in a human body.

Neither silver nor gold interferes with the energy of crystals, and gold enhances the properties of minerals.

Hematite

Hematite is a protection and warrior stone. It enhances the balance of male energies in both men and women.

Jade

Jade is the perfect healing stone and can assist a healing on any malady, physical or spiritual. It is the one stone that enhances the body while drawing negative energy from it. It can and will break when it reaches a point where it has absorbed too much negativity. Most healers should have some jade on their person, in their business, and in their home.

Kyanite

Kyanite is one of the best stones for the cleansing of negativity. It should be one of the stones in your healing room to transform weird energy into positive. It adds to the energy of the healing room and if downloaded with a specific job to do it will become even more powerful. It balances all the other crystals in a room so that the different energies work together.

Unlike most crystals, kyanite never needs to be cleansed. Physically, it takes away stomachache and headaches.

Larimar

Larimar was discovered in the Dominican Republic in 1974. It brings back ancient memories and latent talents and will also transport us to the future and to future talents. It helps to awaken the DNA so we remember divine missions of the past and present.

Moldavite

Moldavite is from a family of stones called tektites. They are the products of meteor impacts, the result of a fusion of heaven and Earth, and so are attractive to metaphysical people as energy stones. They are actually the glass that is formed under the high heat of a meteor as it hits the atmosphere or the Earth itself. They have different colors, depending on the constitution of the meteor blast, the place where it happened, and the composition of the meteor itself. Moldavite is a rare and beautiful green color.

This stone brings the realization that we are connected to All That Is. It is slightly irradiated, so putting it in your home stirs up energy and makes events move faster. This means it is a manifesting stone. It can bring great change to our life. But if we program it to bring us good lessons, we will be able to have a modicum of control over the pace and severity of the lessons learned.

Peridot

Peridot does everything that an emerald does, only to a lesser degree. Many people who can't afford a translucent emerald can afford a clear peridot. Both emerald and peridot enhance our true being.

Pyrite

Pyrite is a stone of protection.

Quartz

Quartz is a strong magnifier of energy, a fact that the ancients intuitively knew and modern science can now fully confirm. Quartz crystals have what modern science calls piezoelectric properties. This means that they are capable of changing a mechanical force into electricity or an electric current into a mechanical force. They have a myriad uses in the modern world, including in electronics, optics, and the manufacture of glass, mortar, grindstones, sandpaper, and cleaning compounds.

Quartz is the second most abundant substance in the Earth. In ancient times quartz crystal clusters would be placed in the four cardinal directions of the home to protect it from negativity of all kinds. The idea was that the negativity would move through the property smoothly, without creating conflict.

Quartz comes in many different colors.

Ruby

People are drawn to the energy of ruby because it enhances courage. Specifically, it gives the wearer the courage to be different and to stand up for what they believe in. This is why so many warriors are drawn to the stone. Ruby also makes the wearer more focused on their goals and the reality they have created. It gives them some spiritual common sense.

Sapphire

Sapphire is any color of the mineral corundum other than red (which is ruby), so comes in many different colors and is as varied as the spectrum of the rainbow. It is an important stone in that it refocuses us on our spiritual path in the highest and best way. It is good for introducing us to our spiritual self.

A sapphire brings us true abundance if we can tolerate its strong energy. Blue sapphire has a stronger energy than the other colors. A good sapphire will realign us constantly, and it's like having a person nagging away, telling you you're out of spiritual and emotional alignment. But when we're in alignment, sapphire enhances our abilities. When we wear it, we can maintain emotional balance when talking to others.

The level of energy a sapphire has differs from stone to stone. The best advice I can give you when buying any expensive gemstone is to know the seller. If a seller tells you that the stone is completely 'natural,' they are likely not telling the truth. Most colored corundum gemstones are either heat-treated or irradiated. This doesn't mean that a particular stone isn't a sapphire or doesn't accelerate energy. But a good energy-accelerator will talk to you and tell in its own language if it wants you to buy it, and you should be able to feel the energy level of the stone when it talks to you in its sacred language.

Smoky Quartz

The coloring of smoky quartz is the result of (natural or artificial) gamma rays and aluminum impurities. The color varies from brown to black and sometimes gray.

Smoky quartz is prized for its ability to transmute negative energy into positive energy. It has a powerful ability to absorb and clear undesirable emotions that have been projected outward. That's why it's a very good stone to have in a therapy room.

Tourmaline

Tourmaline enhances all our spiritual energies. It has the ability to remind us of the beauty of creation.

Turquoise

Turquoise is used for healing the world over, particularly for arthritis. It works as a bridge to connect the material mind and spiritual mind and get them working together.

The Gemstone Saint: Hildegard von Bingen

Our crystal healing traditions come largely from Hildegard von Bingen, a Christian abbess who was born in 1098 in Bermersheim, Germany. She was the first major mystic in German-speaking areas. Her work *Scivias*, describing her religious visions, is still popular today.

The inspiration for Hildegard's work on gemstones, in her medical treatise *Physica*, is thought to be Bishop Marbod of Rennes, who had compiled a book about them 60 years previously. However, others postulate her work to be purely visionary in origin.

Hildegard describes the following 16 healing gems: agate, amethyst, beryl, carnelian, chalcedony, chrysolite, chrysoprase, diamond, hyacinth, jasper, onyx, prase, ruby, sapphire, sardonyx, and topaz. Probably in order to protect her teachings from attack, she didn't offer any blessings directly from the gemstones themselves. So she didn't give them a specific consciousness of their own, but she did suggest that by their very nature they were hostile to evil and intrinsically of God, writing:

> 'Each gem has fire and dampness within it. But the devil shuns,
> hates and despises gemstones because he remembers that
> their beauty appeared in them before he fell from the grace
> accorded to him by God and also because certain gemstones
> are created by fire in which he receives his punishment
> since, by the will of God, he was conquered by fire.'

It would be true to say that the roots of present-day crystal healing reach back to Christian mysticism and it wasn't considered heresy by the medieval Church.

All cultures have used gemstones in much the same way as St Hildegard and, even though separated by thousands of miles, have attributed roughly the same qualities to the same stones. The Native Americans, Chinese, Indians, Egyptians, Romans, Greeks, and Australian Aborigines have all used gemstones for healing. The practice is thousands of years old.

PROGRAMMING INANIMATE OBJECTS

All minerals have the ability to hold memories and can emit energies that have been given to them – programmed into them – by lite thought-forms. Crystals have these abilities *par excellence* and this is the reason, apart from their beauty, why we are so drawn to them as memory-keepers and energy transmitters.

One thing we can do with a crystal is to download the thought-form of Seventh-Plane energy into it and program it with the ability to transmit the energy of that thought-form throughout the house.

One reason why we download stones with a job like this is so that the download overrides any negative memories that are already in them. Another reason is so that the energy we want is fed back to us.

PROGRAM AN INANIMATE OBJECT

1. Go up to the Seventh Plane of Existence (*see pages 13 and 14*) and make the command: 'Creator of All That Is, it is commanded [or requested] that this article be downloaded with the ability of [name ability]. Thank you. It is done, it is done, it is done.'

2. Witness the download going from the Creator into the article.

3. As soon as the process is finished, rinse yourself off in Seventh-Plane energy and stay connected to it.

Energy is fed back to us in a similar way when we place symbolic items in our house or business. Some people have pictures of Jesus or crucifixes that have the deep symbolism of salvation attached to them. Other people put up the 'OM' symbol that represents the sound of the universe. In and of themselves these inorganic symbols have only the power that we instill in them and would have little or no impact without that energy. Nevertheless, this is changing our environment for our benefit.

If you came into my home, you would see that it was a symbol of all the planes of existence. I have stones for the First Plane, fairies and plants for the Second, pictures of my children for the Third, pictures of my ancestors for the Fourth, symbols of the masters for the Fifth, and sacred geometry for the Sixth. This is so that I am reminded that I am part of All That Is.

PROGRAM YOUR ENVIRONMENT TO ENHANCE YOUR LIFE

1. Go up to the Seventh Plane of Existence (see pages 13 and 14) and make the command: 'Creator of All That Is, it is commanded that everything in my environment enhances my life. Thank you. It is done, it is done, it is done.'

2. Witness the articles in your house and surroundings being downloaded with energies that enrich your life.

3. As soon as the process is finished, rinse yourself off in Seventh-Plane energy and stay connected to it.

When you begin to program your surroundings, you may find that there's a lot of 'stuff' that you don't want anymore. Just like your body, your house is a reflection of you. If it is full of clutter, then your mind is full of clutter. If you have clutter on the top of desks, countertops or your refrigerator, you either have young children or a heavy burden in your life. This stems from the feeling that you have to carry the weight of the world on your shoulders. Clean your house and clear your mind! Get rid of anything that's taking energy and not creating energy for you. Don't keep clothes you have no intention of wearing again. Remove everything from your home that isn't serving you. This doesn't mean that you have to buy new furniture, but you should find items that you like and that make you comfortable. If you don't like something, release it! This makes room for abundance.

Charging Your Surroundings

In a Theta state, a condensed thought-form can be instilled in every important article in the home to charge it with the right intentions. Some examples:

- Your kitchen table should be charged that there will always be an abundance of food, and that whoever eats at that table will leave full and satisfied.

- Your walls should allow you to feel safe.

- Your couch should be charged to feel comfortable and inviting.

- Statues and rocks can reflect sacredness and project abundance.

- The bed should be charged with comfort, love, rest, and playfulness.

- Pictures can be charged with nurturing, honor, and inspiration (depending on the theme).

- Carvings can be charged with the appreciation of beauty, majesty, and power.

Charge all the objects in your home and space with your desired intentions. You can have a lot of fun doing this.

You should start with the land beneath you and get rid of any negative soul fragments that have been left behind, and all of the wayward spirits as well.

RELEASING WAYWARDS AND SOUL FRAGMENTS FROM THE EARTH

1. Go up to the Seventh Plane (see pages 13 and 14) and make the command, 'Creator of All That Is, I command that all waywards and negative soul fragments be released from this land. It is done, it is done, it is done. And so it is.'

2. Witness the waywards and soul fragments being sent to God's light.

3. When you've finished, rinse yourself off with Seventh-Plane energy and stay connected to it.

I have a crystal in my house that has the job of getting rid of all the waywards. I have another that has the job of sending positive energy to everyone who comes through the door. Every crystal and even the pictures in my house have a download of a job to do. I call this super *feng shui*. Admittedly, I am a little bit eccentric. I have to drink out of blue cups that are downloaded with: 'Everything that I drink from them is pure and full of energy.'

You should program everything in your house with a specific purpose. One reason for this is that they have ghost imprints from all of the people who've touched them in the past. To an intuitive, this can be a little overwhelming!

Protecting the Home

To protect and enhance the energy that you want in your home, take four crystals, program them accordingly, and put them in the cardinal directions of your property or apartment. This will create vortex energy. The house needs to have a positively charged vortex of energy so you feel rested and energized when you leave.

Once you have created this vortex, as well as programmed objects and decorated your home with crystals, it will have an energy signature all its own and can become a beacon for waywards, spirits, angels, and fairies who are drawn to its light. This is why you should energetically clean your house 20 times a day by putting chimes around it.

Angels and fairies are drawn to chimes, and you should program your house to accept fairy energy, but the fairies must be polite and not mischievous. When you ring a singing bowl, angels and fairies will be drawn to it. Waywards and evil spirits, on the other hand, hate chimes and bells. So putting chimes round your house will stop any negative energy from entering.

As you hang the chimes, download them with: 'Every time you ring, the house and the area are cleansed of negative influences.'

Clocks that have chimes or bells that ring every hour will help inside the house. When I'm away for a long time and there's no one to wind my clocks, I rely on those that are battery-driven and let the chimes do the rest.

Balancing Psychic Abilities

As I mentioned earlier, some intuitive people are naturally inclined to create vortices of energy. Their psychic abilities can also result in wild static electricity. When these kinds of people are emotionally balanced, everything is good. But when they aren't balanced, little technical problems begin to manifest, such as electrical appliances blowing up, lights going out, watches stopping, and so on. At first this is amusing, but after a while it gets expensive. This is why it's important for psychics to maintain their emotional balance.

I learned this years ago when I worked in a potato-processing plant as a quality control technician. I tested the product for sulfides and additives. I would go into the plant to get the test samples and when I walked by the machines, they would simply stop. It didn't take too long for the workers in the plant to notice that it was when I walked by a machine that it broke down.

Potato-factory work is hard, long, and monotonous. So the workers began to call me over to stand by the machine they were operating, so they could take a break from work. When I did stand there, the machine would break down, right on cue. The workers would be chatting for an hour, doing nothing, waiting for it to be fixed.

No machine was beyond me. I could stop the huge potato-flake rollers. I've even stopped X-ray machines when I've been upset.

One day I went over to see my friend Chris, who is also psychic. We had an emotional conversation about life for about an hour and then I left. The next day she called me up and said, 'Vianna, I love you, but maybe we shouldn't get together for a while. When you were over here, between us we blew up my microwave, my television, and my washing machine.'

I remember that when my mother got mad, strange things would happen. One time she got so mad at her boyfriend that all the glasses in the cupboard exploded. This can put a damper on your relationship. The mind is very powerful! If you're blowing things up, it's a good sign that you need to balance your abilities.

Also, as a psychic, you should know that if you're upset or angry you shouldn't get into your car to drive. It's possible that you'll break something electric. You should download anything electric in your life with the program that it's protected from you and it works. And before you use any equipment, you need to be calm. If you get in your car when you're stressed, keep telling yourself that you're balanced. After doing this for a while, you'll get used to this extra psychic energy and problems won't happen as often.

On the other hand, it's possible to heal electrical appliances and other machines. Twenty years ago I had a car that ran on pure love, faith, and prayer. Once I did something that smashed its fuel line. It was so kinked that there was no fuel reaching the engine. When I took the car to the mechanic, he told me he didn't know how it was running at all.

Another time, the car was running rough, so I took it to the mechanic again. He told me that the timing belt had gone out and the spark plugs were gaping so far apart that again he just had no idea how the car was running.

INTERACTING WITH THE LAND

Energy affects us all and so often we don't realize how powerful it is. I think that people are even spontaneously healing and recreating disease in their own body all the time. I think that this has much to do with environmental factors such as the lack of Schumann waves.

The Schumann Waves of the Earth

In 1954 two scientists named Schumann and König reported on their discovery of naturally occurring electromagnetic pulsations on the Earth now called 'Schumann waves.' These are natural waves excited by lightning strikes in the cavity between the surface of the Earth and the ionosphere. The lightning pumps energy into this cavity and causes it to vibrate at extremely low frequencies, creating electromagnetic waves that travel around the Earth at the speed of light, circumnavigating the globe an average of 7.83 times per second.

A physician, Dr. Ankermueller, realized that this frequency correlated with the average frequency of alpha brainwaves in humans and concluded that the Schumann waves were in essence the 'thought-waves' of the Earth. He contacted Professor Schumann, who arranged for one of his doctorate candidates, Herbert König, to look into it. He compared human EEG recordings with electromagnetic fields in the environment and was able to show that Schumann waves were actually very close to the frequency of alpha rhythms.

Later research by Dr. Wolfgang Ludwig found that man-made electromagnetic signals within the atmosphere made the accurate measurement of Schumann waves almost impossible in a city. In space, when the first cosmonauts and astronauts were not exposed to Schumann waves at all, they reported emotional distress and migraines.

But even though our cities are interrupting the All That Is rhythm of the Schumann waves of the Earth, we can tell our spirits to create them and this will compensate for the lack of them.

The Land Heals Us

We interact with the Earth in so many ways. Many healers have an overwhelming need to heal the Earth of the pollution we've caused since the advent of the industrial revolution. While this is very important, we should understand that the Earth heals us as well.

The Earth has recorded all the events that have taken place here. While there is an imprint of sadness in these stored memories and many psychics feel it, this doesn't mean the land has a need for us to heal her. She will heal herself from all the mistakes that we are making with regard to our environment. The Earth is so old that the cycle of destruction and rebirth has happened many times before. We are limited in our understanding of how powerful a healer our Mother Earth truly is because of the short lifespan of our physical bodies. But as immortal spirits, we will see a time when the Earth is reborn and nature restores itself to balance. We may destroy our environment, but the Earth will go on. Life, death, and rebirth are natural processes of the Earth. That is the divine cycle.

This doesn't mean, however, that we shouldn't take action to change the way we use our resources in the *now*. We must take direct action so that we don't destroy the environment and this existence.

Remember that given the chance, the land will heal itself, and it is this healing energy that we should focus on, not the sadness and guilt we feel. If we can accept the healing energy of the Earth, the Earth herself will grow stronger.

As we send healing energy to the land, we have to be able to accept healing energy back from it. Even a houseplant that is loved too much will die if we send a barrage of love to it without receiving love from it. If you ask, the Earth will send you healing energy. You'll be surprised if you open up and receive it.

Focus on letting the land heal you as much as you focus on healing the land. The land *will* heal you, but only if you aren't too busy trying to heal it. The more energy you put into healing the land, the more sadness you'll bring up, because there are layers and layers of sadness in the land. If you concentrate on it, you won't be able to move forward. Instead, send love to the land and accept the love that comes back. This will create a divine cycle between humanity and the Earth.

Ancient tribal cultures followed this divine cycle and some elements of it survive to this day. Native Americans still know about accepting love from the Earth. It is in the ancestral memories of their DNA. The Australian aborigines know the psychic truth of letting the land guide them, and that they do not guide the soul of the land.

The soul of the Earth is timeless. I asked the Creator when the end of this world would come and I saw it would be long after we'd gone. I saw that we might destroy ourselves, but after a few thousand years the Earth would be refreshed and life would go on without us. Now that the masters have come to the Third Plane, the chances of avoiding destruction and changing this planet to a vibration of love have moved up to 65 percent. However, these percentages move up and down according to the daily choices we're making. On some level we're aware of this. When things are changing in a positive way, we feel physically good. But when our chances of saving ourselves go down, it's likely that we'll have some aches and pains we didn't have before.

Up until now, as a species we've been on overdrive to do anything to survive, even at the cost of the very thing that gives us life: our environment. The challenge that we have is to overcome these ancient self-destructive programs.

Unfortunately, we seem hardwired to create destruction and war. There's always the threat of war someplace on the planet. This propensity toward conflict has left memories in the Earth as well as a collective consciousness in our species that must be overcome in order for us to survive. If we obsess about the threat of war, the people who were killed in the past, and the anguish and destruction that are the face of war, then this form of consciousness will pervade our society.

Stop being afraid of war, desolation, negativity, and hatred. Let the positive energy of the Earth in to heal you. Go up and connect to the All That Is and say, 'I am open to whatever love the world wants to give me,' and the negative memories of the Earth will not affect you.

RECEIVING HEALING FROM THE EARTH

1. Go up to the Seventh Plane of Existence (*see pages 13 and 14*) and make the command: *'Creator of All That Is, it is commanded [or requested] that Mother Earth heals me and I accept it. Thank you. It is done, it is done, it is done.'*

2. Witness the healing energy coming into your space.

3. When you have finished, rinse yourself off with Seventh-Plane energy and stay connected to it.

Blessings from the Land – Blessings Are Stronger Than Curses

When Guy and I first got together, he wanted to fix up his old house rather than leave it, because he loved it so much. He promised me that he'd put an addition on and fix it up. I agreed, but I found the house had a lot of challenges! Some of these included heating systems and water purification. In time, we made the addition – and renovations too numerous to mention.

By the time it was finished, I'd made a darling little country cottage out of it. However, no matter how much we renovated the house, it didn't seem that it was mine. I programmed it, I took curses off it – you name it, I tried it. Each time I'd do clearings on it, there'd be memories coming up from the previous owners. Some of these were from Guy's ex-wife and from the arguments that had gone on in that house.

I had a hard time figuring it out, but one day I walked into the house and realized it was *Guy's* memories that I was feeling. It wasn't the house at all; it was Guy and his feelings about it.

One day I looked at my husband and said, 'You know, I love you, but I'm moving.'

Guy told me he wasn't going to move unless he had trees. So we manifested what we wanted and we found a house with thousands of trees in only a week.

Then we had to sell the old house. At first, it wouldn't sell because Guy was still holding on to it. So I went out of my space to see if there was any kind of energy that was holding him to the land by way of a curse. I found out that instead of it being a *curse* that held him to the land, it was a *blessing* that was holding him. This was because the land had bestowed a blessing on him as its caretaker. With Guy's permission, I removed the blessing and allowed the land to bless another caretaker. After that it was easy for him to move on with his life.

Within a week, we'd sold the old house. Several months later, I was driving by it and I could feel that it didn't like its present caretaker. Directly after that, it was sold to a country person who understood how to take care of a house in the country. I could tell that the house was happy once again.

The new house we'd bought was waiting for me to be its caretaker. It had been on the market for a year and hadn't sold. When I first viewed it, I could tell that this was because when people came to look at it, the teenage girl who was living there would scare them away, or the spirit of her father, who had committed suicide in the house, would haunt them. However, this didn't scare me, so we went to look at it again.

The second time I viewed the house, I was left alone in it for a while. The voice of the house told me to go upstairs and look on a desk that was up there. On the desk there was a paper. On the paper, it said how much the woman who owned the house had purchased it for, which was very different than what she was asking for it (which was astronomical). I knew then what I could offer to get her to sell the house. I made two offers, and she took the second. You see, objects, houses, all sorts of things have feelings of their own, and you should be aware that you might be blessed to be their caretaker.

The land itself lays an enchantment over the people who own it. The earth, the plants and trees and the animals of the land all combine their energies to ensure they're properly taken care of. In and of itself, this isn't a bad thing if the owner is aware of it. But some land will literally work its owner into oblivion. There should be a healthy relationship between land and owner. Any energy that you send to a plant is reflected back to you and magnified. If you're sending out love to the land, it should reflect it back to you. If it does then you won't be sucked dry by the correspondence.

Concerning curses, sometimes what we perceive to be a curse is only another person's negative thoughts. I believe that people can become so sensitive that they hear other people's negative thoughts and perceive them to be a curse directed at them. In any event, blessings are stronger than curses, oaths or vows. If you bless yourself, it will protect you from a curse. (If you aren't able to do that, there may be genetic programs in place because of past superstitions. Energy test for this.)

In order to release a blessing from the land, use the following exercise.

RELEASING A BLESSING FROM THE LAND

1. Go up to the Seventh Plane of Existence (*see pages 13 and 14*) and make the command: *'Creator of All That Is, it is commanded [or requested] that I am released from this blessing, this enchantment, from this land. Thank you. It is done, it is done, it is done.'*

2. Witness the energy of the enchantment being sent to God's light.

3. Once you have finished, rinse yourself off with Seventh-Plane energy and stay connected to it.

4. Now take a picture of the land.

BRING IT ALL TOGETHER

This final exercise will guide you on a journey to feel, taste, touch, and see the different planes. Through this experience, you can expand your awareness to bring all the planes together and discover that *you* are the planes of existence.

EXPERIENCE ALL THE PLANES OF EXISTENCE

1. Go up to the Seventh Plane of Existence (*see pages 13 and 14*) and make the command: *'Creator of All That Is, It is commanded [or requested] to travel to each plane of existence, to feel, touch, taste, and experience each in all its glory, on this [month, day, year, time]. Thank you. It is done, it is done, it is done.'*

2. Visualize your consciousness being sent to the First Plane of Existence.

3. Connect to the minerals from the First Plane of Existence and how they heal. The First Plane is the minerals, the crystals, the soil, and the rocks. It is every piece of the Earth, from the smallest crystal to the largest mountain, in inorganic form. Experience the crystals and their energy.

4. Connect to the Second Plane of Existence and feel the power of herbal medicines. The Second Plane consists of organic material: vitamins, plants, trees, and elementals.

5. Connect to the Third Plane of Existence and perceive the illusion. The Third Plane consists of protein-based molecules, carbon-based structures, and amino acid-based chains. These organic compounds are the basis of life on this plane.

6. Connect to the Fourth Plane of Existence and your ancestors. The Fourth Plane is the realm of spirit.

7. Connect to the Fifth Plane of Existence and the masters. The Fifth Plane is plane of the angels, the Council of Twelve, our soul families, the masters, our heavenly father, and our heavenly mother.

8. Contact to the Sixth Plane of Existence and the Laws.

9. Bring the knowledge of all these planes within yourself and know you are the planes of existence.

10. When you have finished, rinse yourself off with Seventh-Plane energy and stay connected to that divine energy.

Appendix

THE FIVE STEPS OF BELIEF WORK AND THE EIGHT WAYS OF DIGGING

THE FIVE STEPS OF BELIEF WORK

The five steps are as follows:

1. Establish a bond of trust with the other person that will encourage open communication.

2. Identify the issue that the person wants to work on.

3. Begin the digging process. This is the search for the bottom belief that will release all the beliefs stacked above it.

4. Go up and connect to the Creator and witness the beliefs being changed on the four levels of belief – the core, genetic, history, and soul levels.

5. Confirm that the beliefs have been released and replaced by energy testing.

THE EIGHT WAYS OF DIGGING

Digging work is knowing how to ask the right questions and to identify the underlying bottom belief that will release all the beliefs that created it. There are eight common approaches to digging work.

1. Basic Questions

These are:

'Who?'

'What?'

'Where?'

'Why?'

'How?'

Examples:

'Why do you think so?'

'What did you learn from it?'

'How did it serve you?'

If the person says, 'I don't know,' ask, 'What if you did know?' or 'But if you did know...?' This is an opening to deeper belief-programs.

2. Phobias

Identify the deepest fear that underlies all other fears. Ask:

'What is the worst thing that could happen if you were in a given situation?'

'What would happen next in that situation?'

3. Drama (Trauma)

- Identify an incident in the past that first evoked the traumatic emotions, such as anger, sadness, resentment, guilt, and refusal.

- Then identify the current indicators of the feelings of the person:

  'When did you begin to feel that way?'

  'Whom do you feel that way towards?'

  'Where were you when you began to feel that way?'

'What was happening at that time?'

'How do you feel about the situation?'

'What action would you like to take from the feelings you are having about the situation?'

- Identify when the feeling evolved:

  'When was the first time you were in a similar situation and experienced a similar feeling?'

  'How did you feel then?'

- Witness the beliefs being released and changed on the four levels of belief, (core, genetic, history, and soul).

- Download the feelings that are needed to help the person to recognize the bottom belief.

- Ask:

  'What did you learn from that experience?'

  'Why did you have to experience that?'

  'How did it serve you and how does it continue to serve you?'

4. Sickness

- Find out what the issues are and then start digging deeper.

- Find out why the person became sick:

  'When did the illness start?'

  'What was going on in your life at that time?'

- Find out why the person remains sick:

  'What was the best thing that happened to you as a result of being sick?'

  'What did you learn from being sick?'

- Find out why the person cannot heal:

  'What would happen if you were healed completely?'

5. Manifesting

- Ask the client to visualize what they would do if they had all the money they needed.

- Ask the client where they would be if they had all the money they wanted.

- How does the individual feel with all the money they ever wanted?

- Is there a significant other in the person's life, and if there is, how does the person's family/friends/soul mate react to all that money, and so forth? Discover issues that make the client uncomfortable in their visualization and start digging deeper to resolve these issues. Ask:

  'What would you do if you had all the money you ever wanted?'

  'What could go wrong in that situation?'

6. Gene work

If you find, by muscle testing, that the person has certain beliefs but they do not consciously believe in them, you may find that they become confused, making it difficult to continue your digging work. Their beliefs may be their ancestor's genetic beliefs that have been passed down to them. Ask the following questions and continue digging:

  'Is this your mother's belief?'

  'Is this your father's belief?'

  'Is this your ancestor's belief?'

7. Group consciousness beliefs

When many people have the same belief, they accept it as a fact and it becomes a group consciousness belief. Extract these beliefs and completely eliminate them so that the client can continue.

Examples:

'Diabetes is incurable.'

'I am afraid of using my power.'

'I took a vow of poverty.'

Downloads:

'Diabetes is curable.'

'I can use my power safely and peacefully.'

'The vow of poverty is completely ended.'

8. The impossible

This work is performed not to find blocks but to reprogram your brain to accept what is perceived as impossible. Ask:

'What would happen if...?'

This Appendix was compiled by Hiroyuki Miyazaki from the teachings of Vianna Stibal.

RESOURCES

ThetaHealing Seminars

ThetaHealing is an energy-healing modality founded by Vianna Stibal, with certified instructors around the world. The seminars and books of ThetaHealing are designed as a therapeutic self-help guide to develop the ability of the mind to heal. ThetaHealing includes the following seminars and books:

ThetaHealing® seminars taught by certified ThetaHealing® instructors:

ThetaHealing Basic DNA 1 and 2 Practitioner Seminar

ThetaHealing Advanced DNA 2½ Practitioner Seminar

ThetaHealing Manifesting and Abundance Practitioner Seminar

ThetaHealing Intuitive Anatomy Practitioner Seminar

ThetaHealing Rainbow Children Practitioner Seminar

ThetaHealing Disease and Disorders Practitioner Seminar

ThetaHealing World Relations Practitioner Seminar

ThetaHealing DNA 3 Practitioner Seminar

ThetaHealing Animal Practitioner Seminar

ThetaHealing Dig Deeper Practitioner Seminar

ThetaHealing Plant Practitioner Seminar

ThetaHealing SoulMate Practitioner Seminar

ThetaHealing Rhythm Practitioner Seminar

ThetaHealing Planes of Existence Practitioner Seminar

Certification seminars taught exclusively by Vianna at the ThetaHealing® Institute of Knowledge:

ThetaHealing Basic DNA 1 and 2 Instructors' Seminar

ThetaHealing Advanced DNA 2½ Instructors' Seminar

ThetaHealing Manifesting and Abundance Instructors' Seminar

ThetaHealing Intuitive Anatomy Instructors' Seminar

ThetaHealing Rainbow Children Instructors' Seminar

ThetaHealing Disease and Disorders Instructors' Seminar

ThetaHealing World Relations Instructors' Seminar

ThetaHealing DNA 3 Instructors' Seminar

ThetaHealing Animal Instructors' Seminar

ThetaHealing Dig Deeper Instructors' Seminar

ThetaHealing Plant Instructors' Seminar

ThetaHealing SoulMate Instructors' Seminar

ThetaHealing Rhythm Instructors' Seminar

ThetaHealing Planes of Existence Instructors' Seminar

ThetaHealing is always growing and expanding, and new courses are added often.

Books:

ThetaHealing® (Hay House, 2006, 2010)

Advanced ThetaHealing® (Hay House, 2011)

ThetaHealing® Diseases and Disorders (Hay House, 2012)

On the Wings of Prayer (Hay House, 2012)

ThetaHealing® Rhythm for Finding Your Perfect Weight (Hay House, 2013)

ABOUT THE AUTHOR

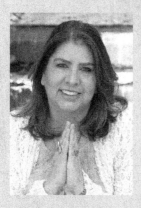

Vianna Stibal is a young grandmother, an artist and a writer. Her natural charisma and compassion for those in need of help have also led to her being known as a healer, intuitive, and teacher.

After being taught how to connect with the Creator to co-create and facilitate the unique process called ThetaHealing, Vianna knew that she must share this gift with as many people as she could. It was this love and appreciation for the Creator and humanity that allowed her to develop the ability to see clearly into the human body and witness many instant healings.

Her encyclopaedic knowledge of the body's systems and deep understanding of the human psyche, based on her own experience as well as the insight given to her by the Creator, makes Vianna the perfect practitioner of this amazing technique. She has worked successfully with such medical challenges as hepatitis C, Epstein-Barr virus, AIDS, herpes, various types of cancers and many other disorders, diseases, and genetic defects.

Vianna knows that the ThetaHealing technique is teachable, but beyond that she knows that it needs to be taught. She conducts seminars all over the world to teach people of all races, beliefs, and religions. She has trained teachers and practitioners who are working in 152 countries, but her work will not stop there! She is committed to spreading this healing paradigm throughout the world.

www.thetahealing.com

251

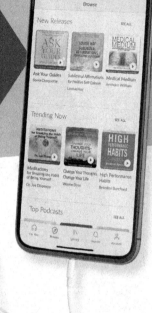

We hope you enjoyed this Hay House book. If you'd like to receive our online catalog featuring additional information on Hay House books and products, or if you'd like to find out more about the Hay Foundation, please contact:

Hay House LLC, P.O. Box 5100, Carlsbad, CA 92018-5100
(760) 431-7695 or (800) 654-5126
www.hayhouse.com® • www.hayfoundation.org

Published in Australia by:
Hay House Australia Publishing Pty Ltd
18/36 Ralph St., Alexandria NSW 2015
Phone: +61 (02) 9669 4299
www.hayhouse.com.au

Published in the United Kingdom by:
Hay House UK Ltd
The Sixth Floor, Watson House,
54 Baker Street, London W1U 7BU
Phone: +44 (0) 203 927 7290
www.hayhouse.co.uk

Published in India by:
Hay House Publishers (India) Pvt Ltd
Muskaan Complex, Plot No. 3,
B-2, Vasant Kunj, New Delhi 110 070
Phone: +91 11 41761620
www.hayhouse.co.in

Let Your Soul Grow

Experience life-changing transformation—one video at a time—with guidance from the world's leading experts.

www.healyourlifeplus.com